Affordable Keto Air Fryer Diet Cookbook

Tasty and Delicious Recipes to boost your Health and Effortless your Metabolism

River Hunt

Table of Contents

Ginger-Garlic Swordfish with Mushrooms

Cook Time:

15 minutes

Servings:3

Ingredients:

1 pound swordfish steak

1 teaspoon ginger-garlic paste

Sea salt and ground black pepper, to taste

1/4 teaspoon cayenne pepper

1/4 teaspoon dried dill weed

1/2 pound mushrooms

Directions:

1.Rub the swordfish steak with ginger-garlic paste; season with salt, black pepper, cayenne pepper and dried dill.

2.Spritz the fish with a nonstick cooking spray and transfer to the Air Fryer cooking basket. Cook at 400 degrees F for 5 minutes.

3.Now, add the mushrooms to the cooking basket and continue to cook for 5 minutes longer until tender and fragrant. Eat warm. Enjoy!

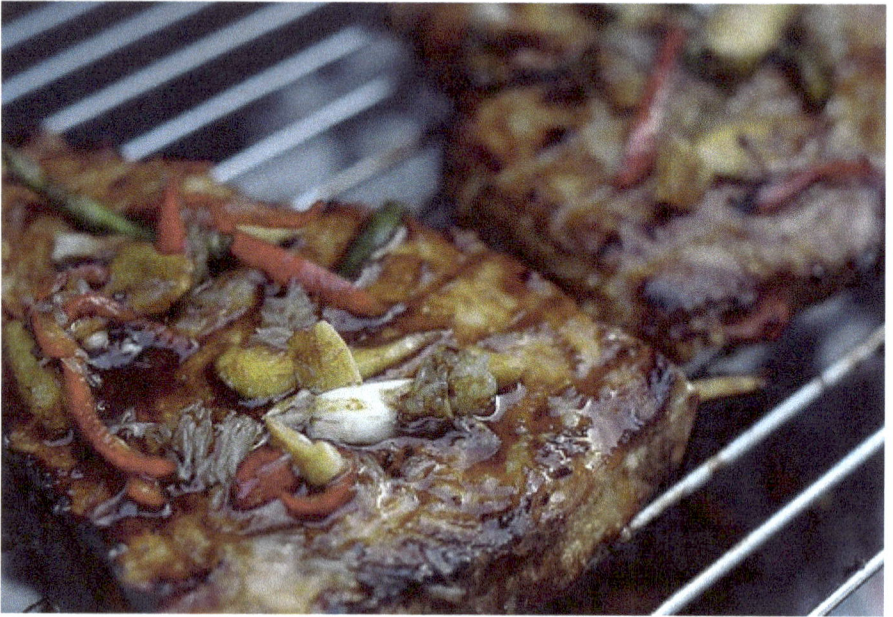

Melt-in-Your Mouth Salmon with Cilantro Sauce

Cook Time:

15 minutes

Servings:2

Ingredients:

1 pound salmon fillets

1 teaspoon coconut oil

Sea salt and ground black pepper, to season

2 heaping tablespoons cilantro

1/2 cup Mexican crema

1 tablespoon fresh lime juice

Directions:

1.Rinse and pat your salmon dry using paper towels. Toss the salmon with coconut oil, salt and black pepper.

2.Cook the salmon filets in your Air Fryer at 380 degrees F for 6 minutes; turn the salmon filets over and cook on the other side for 6 to 7 minutes.

3.Meanwhile, mix the remaining ingredients in your blender or food processor. Spoon the cilantro sauce over the salmon filets and serve immediately.

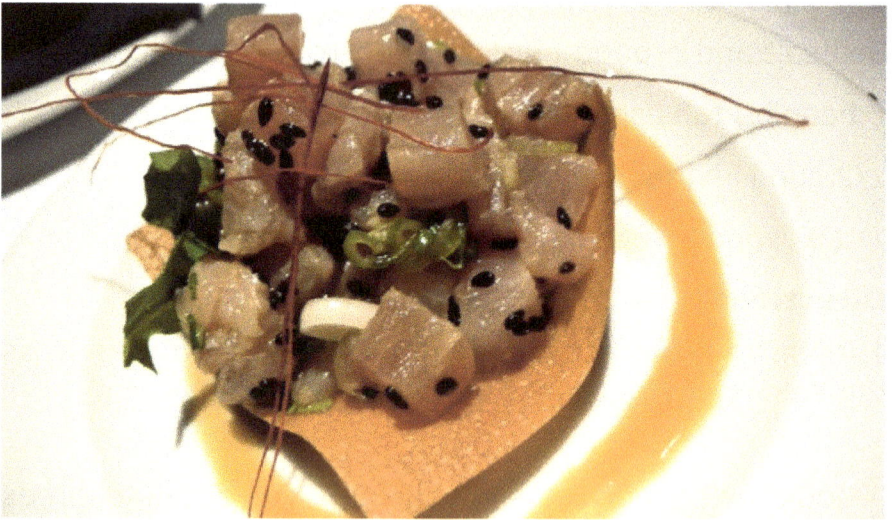

Salmon with Baby Bok Choy

Cook Time:

20 minutes

Servings:3

Ingredients:

1 pound salmon filets

1 teaspoon garlic chili paste

1 teaspoon sesame oil

1 tablespoon honey

1 tablespoon soy sauce

1 pound baby Bok choy, bottoms removed

Kosher salt and black pepper, to taste

Directions:

1.Start by preheating your Air Fryer to 380 degrees F. Toss the salmon fillets with garlic chili paste, sesame oil, honey, soy sauce, salt and black pepper.

2.Cook the salmon in the preheated Air Fryer for 6 minutes; turn the filets over and cook an additional 6 minutes.

3.Then, cook the baby Bok choy at 350 degrees F for 3 minutes; shake the basket and cook an additional 3 minutes. Salt and pepper to taste.

4.Serve the salmon fillets with the roasted baby Bok choy. Enjoy!

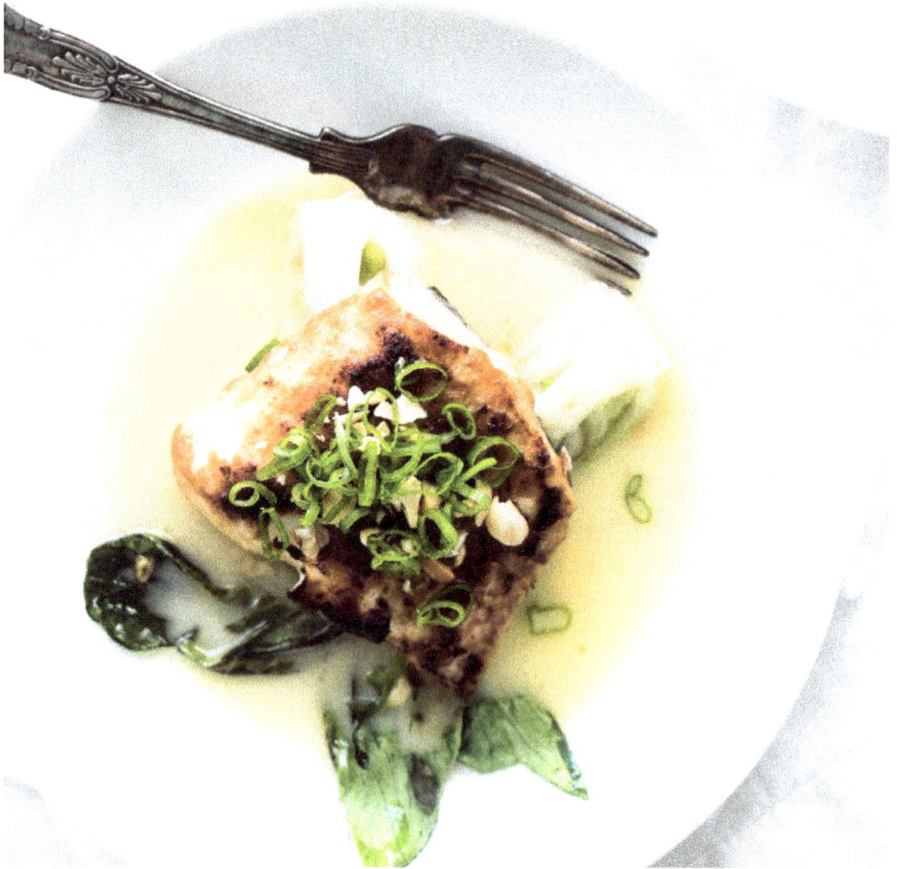

Crispy Tilapia Fillets

Cook Time:

20 minutes

Servings:5

Ingredients:

5 tablespoons all-purpose flour

Sea salt and white pepper, to taste

1 teaspoon garlic paste

2 tablespoons extra virgin olive oil

1/2 cup cornmeal

5 tilapia fillets, slice into halves

Directions:

1.Combine the flour, salt, white pepper, garlic paste, olive oil, and cornmeal in a Ziploc bag. Add the fish fillets and shake to coat well.

2.Spritz the Air Fryer basket with cooking spray. Cook in the preheated Air Fryer at 400 degrees F for 10 minutes; turn them over and cook for 6 minutes more.

3.Work in batches. Serve with lemon wedges if desired. Enjoy!

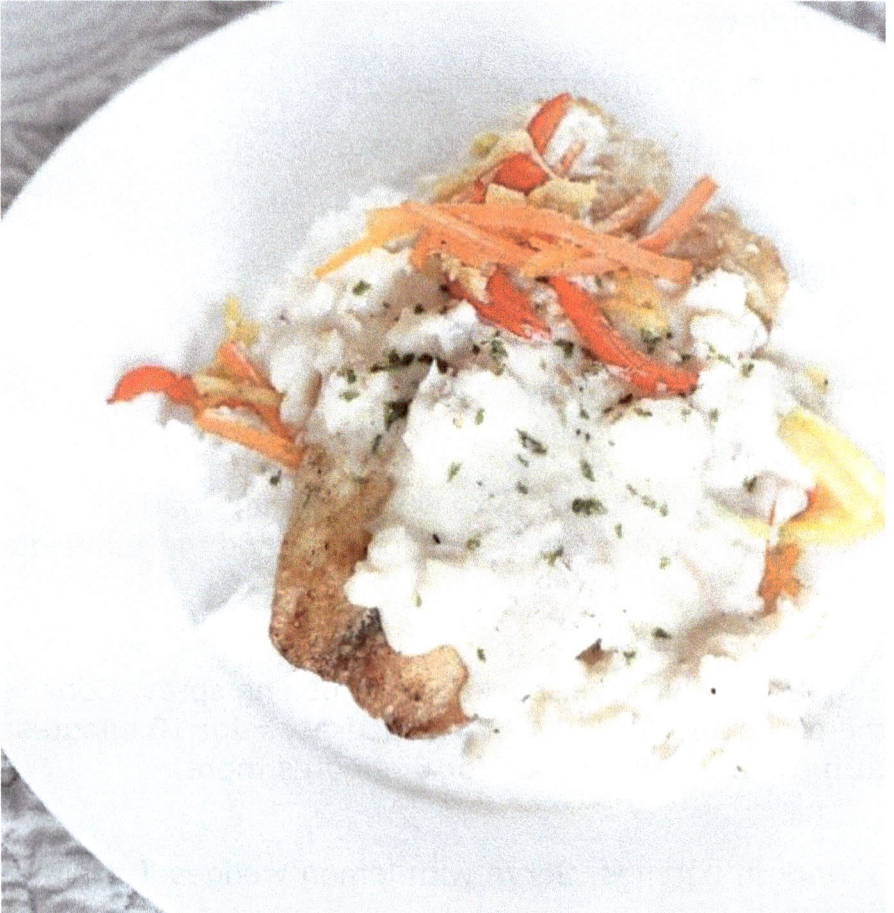

Easy Prawns Parmigiana

Cook Time:

20 minutes

Servings:4

Ingredients:

2 egg whites

1 cup all-purpose flour

1 cup Parmigiano-Reggiano, grated

1/2 cup fine breadcrumbs

1/2 teaspoon celery seeds

1/2 teaspoon porcini powder

1/2 teaspoon onion powder

1 teaspoon garlic powder

1/2 teaspoon dried rosemary

1/2 teaspoon sea salt

1/2 teaspoon ground black pepper

1 ½ pounds prawns, deveined

Directions:

1.To make a breading station, whisk the egg whites in a shallow dish.

2.In a separate dish, place the all-purpose flour. In a third dish, thoroughly combine the Parmigiano-Reggiano, breadcrumbs, and seasonings; mix to combine well.

3.Dip the prawns in the flour, then, into the egg whites; lastly, dip them in the parm/breadcrumb mixture.

4.Roll until they are covered on all sides. Cook in the preheated Air Fryer at 390 degrees F for 5 to 7 minutes or until golden brown. Work in batches.

5.Serve with lemon wedges if desired. Enjoy!

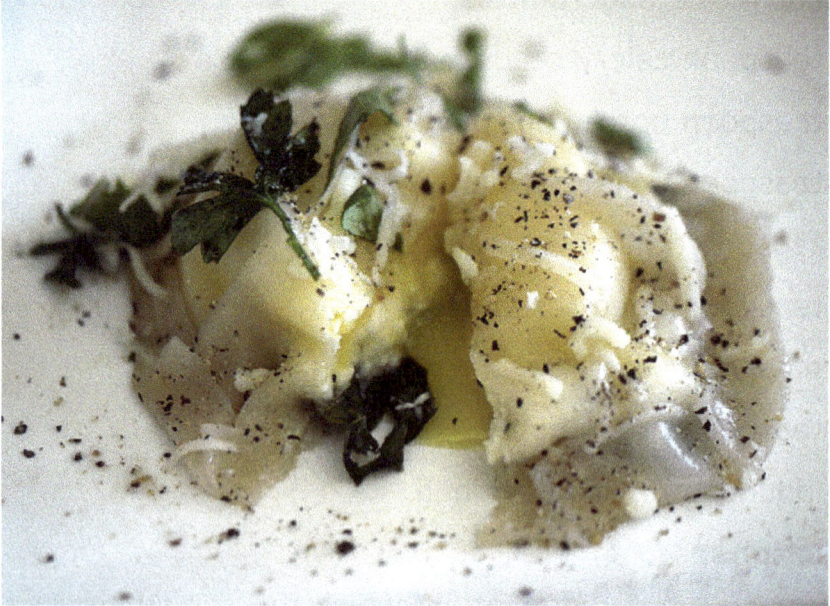

Greek-Style Roast Fish

Cook Time:

20 minutes

Servings:3

Ingredients:

2 tablespoons olive oil

1 red onion, sliced

2 cloves garlic, chopped

1 Florina pepper, deveined and minced

3 pollock fillets, skinless

2 ripe tomatoes, diced

12 Kalamata olives, pitted and chopped

2 tablespoons capers

1 teaspoon oregano

1 teaspoon rosemary

Sea salt, to taste

1/2 cup white wine

Directions:

1.Start by preheating your Air Fryer to 360 degrees F. Heat the oil in a baking pan.

2.Once hot, sauté the onion, garlic, and pepper for 2 to 3 minutes or until fragrant. Add the fish fillets to the baking pan.

3.Top with the tomatoes, olives, and capers. Sprinkle with the oregano, rosemary, and salt.

4.Pour in white wine and transfer to the cooking basket. Turn the temperature to 395 degrees F and bake for 10 minutes.

5.Taste for seasoning and serve on individual plates, garnished with some extra Mediterranean herbs if desired. Enjoy!

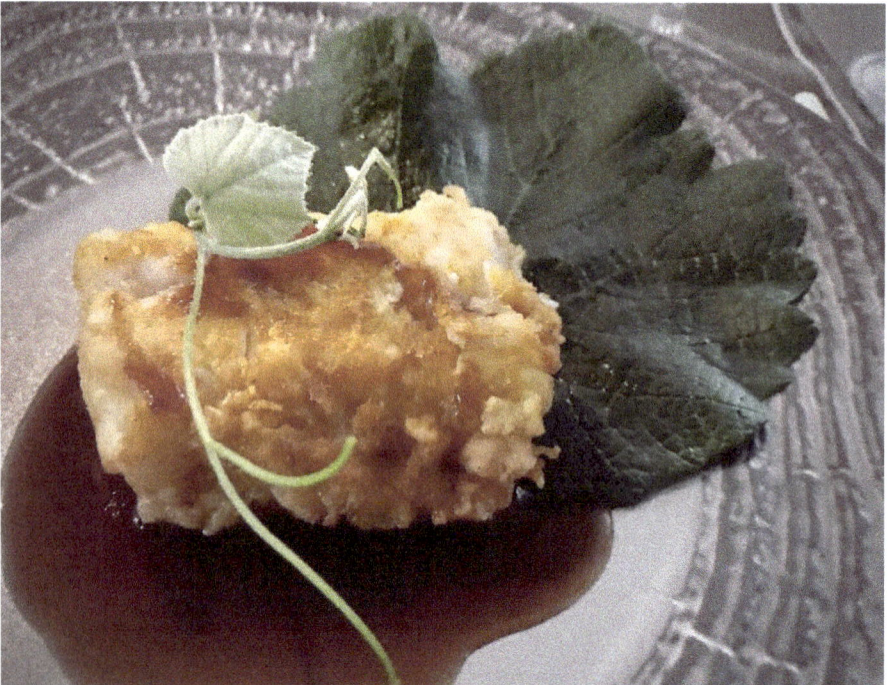

Filet of Flounder Cutlets

Cook Time:

15 minutes

Servings:3

Ingredients:

1 egg

1/2 cup cracker crumbs

1/2 cup Pecorino Romano cheese, grated

Sea salt and white pepper, to taste

1/2 teaspoon cayenne pepper

1 teaspoon dried parsley flakes

2 flounder fillets

Directions:

1.To make a breading station, whisk the egg until frothy. In another bowl, mix the cracker crumbs, Pecorino Romano cheese, and spices.

2.Dip the fish in the egg mixture and turn to coat evenly; then, dredge in the cracker crumb mixture, turning a couple of times to coat evenly.

3.Cook in the preheated Air Fryer at 390 degrees F for 5 minutes; turn them over and cook another 5 minutes. Enjoy!

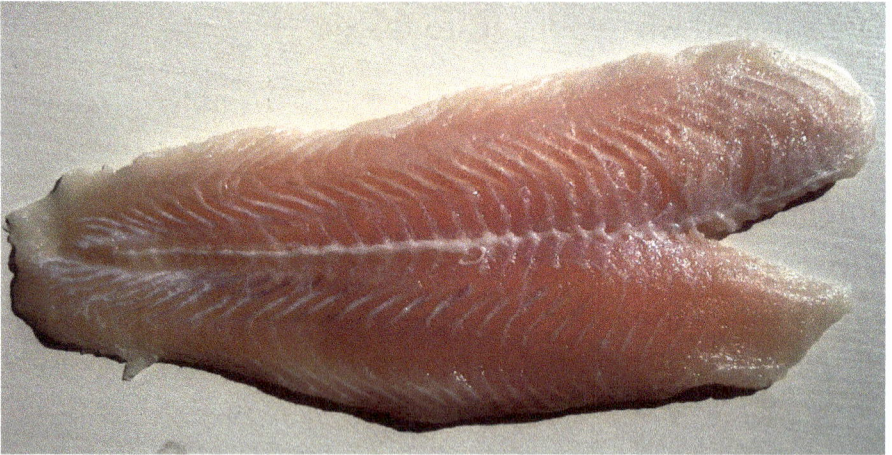

Orange Glazed Scallops

Cook Time:

15 minutes

Servings: 3

Ingredients:

1 pound jumbo sea scallops

1 tablespoon soy sauce

2 tablespoons orange juice

1 teaspoon orange zest

1/2 teaspoon fresh parsley, minced

1 tablespoon olive oil

Sea salt, to taste

1/2 teaspoon ground black pepper

Directions:

1.Start by preheating your Air Fryer to 400 degrees F. Toss all ingredients in mixing bowl.

2.Place the scallops in the lightly greased cooking basket and cook for 7 minutes, shaking the basket halfway through the cooking time.

3.Work in batches. Taste, adjust the seasonings and serve warm. Enjoy!

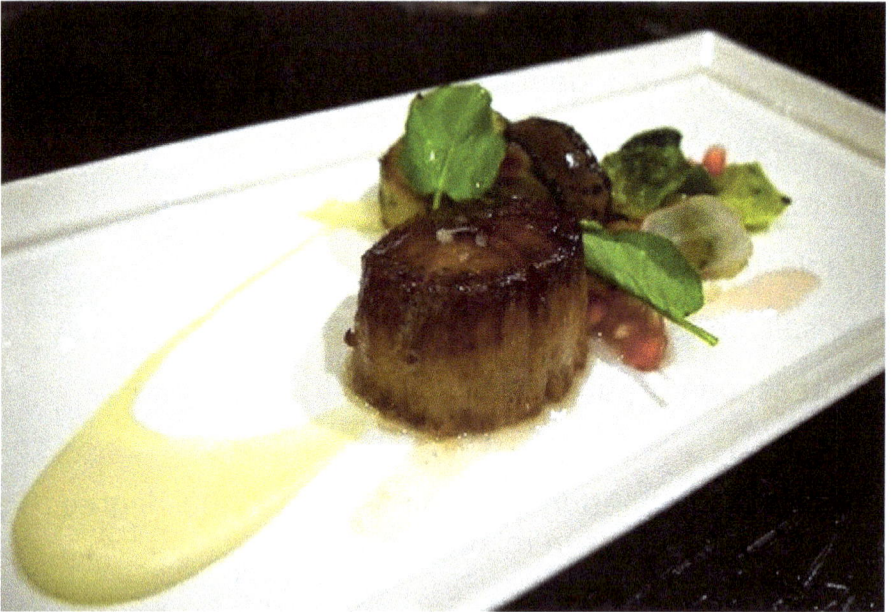

Jamaican-Style Fish and Potato Fritters

Cook Time:

30 minutes

Servings: 2

Ingredients:

1/2 pound sole fillets

1/2 pound mashed potatoes

1 egg, well beaten

1/2 cup red onion, chopped

2 garlic cloves, minced

2 tablespoons fresh parsley, chopped

1 bell pepper, finely chopped

1/2 teaspoon scotch bonnet pepper, minced

1 tablespoon olive oil

1 tablespoon coconut aminos

1/2 teaspoon paprika

Salt and white pepper, to taste

Directions:

1. Start by preheating your Air Fryer to 395 degrees F. Spritz the sides and bottom of the cooking basket with cooking spray.

2. Cook the sole fillets in the preheated Air Fryer for 10 minutes, flipping them halfway through the cooking time.

3.In a mixing bowl, mash the sole fillets into flakes. Stir in the remaining ingredients. Shape the fish mixture into patties.

4.Bake in the preheated Air Fryer at 390 degrees F for 14 minutes, flipping them halfway through the cooking time. Serve and enjoy!

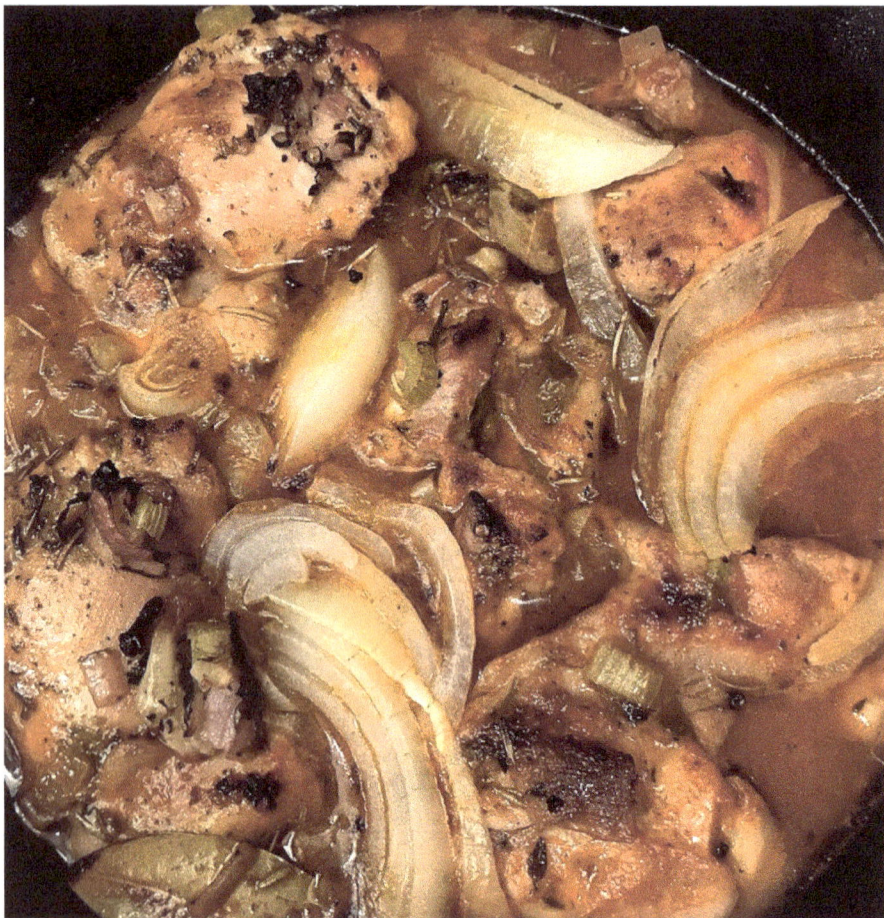

Salmon Fillets with Herbs and Garlic

Cook Time:

15 minutes

Servings:3

Ingredients:

1 pound salmon fillets

Sea salt and ground black pepper, to taste

1 tablespoon olive oil

1 sprig thyme

2 sprigs rosemary

2 cloves garlic, minced

1 lemon, sliced

Directions:

1.Pat the salmon fillets dry and season them with salt and pepper; drizzle salmon fillets with olive oil and place in the Air Fryer cooking basket.

2.Cook the salmon fillets at 380 degrees F for 7 minutes; turn them over, top with thyme, rosemary and garlic and continue to cook for 5 minutes more.

3.Serve topped with lemon slices and enjoy

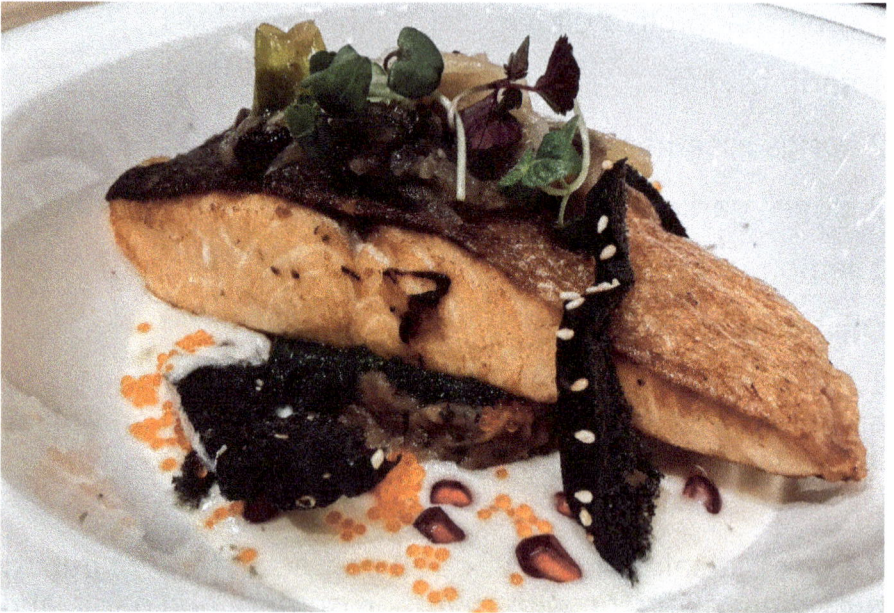

Garlic Butter Scallops

Cook Time:

10 minutes

Servings: 3

Ingredients:

1/2 pound scallops

Coarse sea salt and ground black pepper, to taste

1/4 teaspoon cayenne pepper

1/4 teaspoon dried oregano

1/4 teaspoon dried basil

2 tablespoons butter pieces, cold

1 teaspoon garlic, minced

1 teaspoon lemon zest

Directions:

1.Sprinkle the scallops with salt, black pepper, cayenne pepper, oregano and basil.

2.Spritz your scallops with a nonstick cooking oil and transfer them to the Air Fryer cooking basket.

3.Cook the scallops at 400 degrees F for 6 to 7 minutes, shaking the basket halfway through the cooking time.

4.In the meantime, melt the butter in a small saucepan over medium-high heat.

5.Once hot, add in the garlic and continue to sauté until fragrant, about 1 minute.

6.Add in lemon zest, taste and adjust the seasonings. Spoon the garlic butter over the warm scallops and serve. Enjoy!

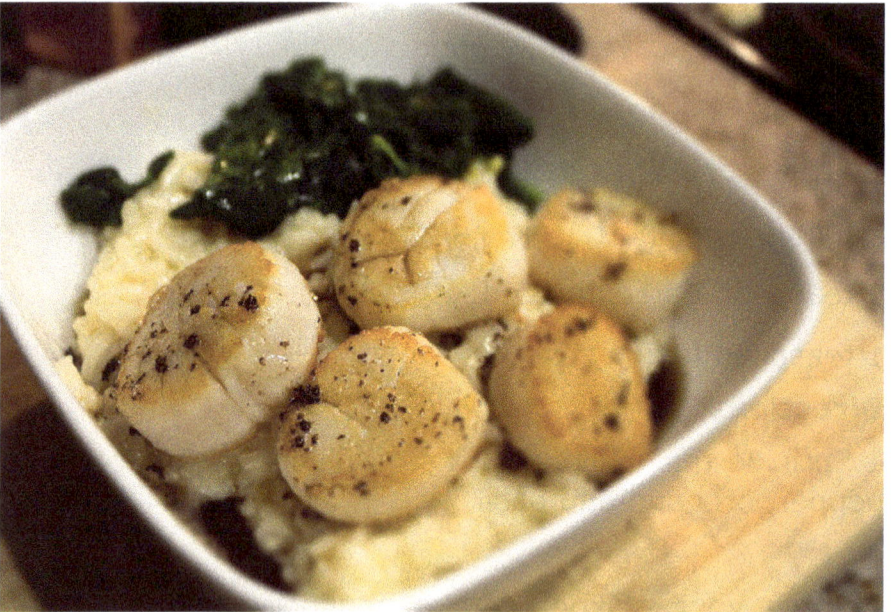

Ahi Tuna with Peppers and Tartare Sauce

Cook Time:

15 minutes

Servings: 2

Ingredients:

2 ahi tuna steaks

2 Spanish peppers, quartered

1 teaspoon olive oil

1/2 teaspoon garlic powder

Salt and freshly ground black pepper, to taste

Tartare sauce:

4 tablespoons mayonnaise

2 tablespoons sour cream

1 tablespoon baby capers, drained

1 tablespoon gherkins, drained and chopped

2 tablespoons white onion, minced

Directions:

1.Pat the ahi tuna dry using kitchen towels. Toss the ahi tuna and Spanish peppers with olive oil, garlic powder, salt and black pepper.

2.Cook the ahi tuna and peppers in the preheated Air Fryer at 400 degrees F for 10 minutes, flipping them halfway through the cooking time.

3.Meanwhile, whisk all the sauce ingredients until well combined.

4.Plate the ahi tuna steaks and arrange Spanish peppers around them. Serve with tartare sauce on the side and enjoy!

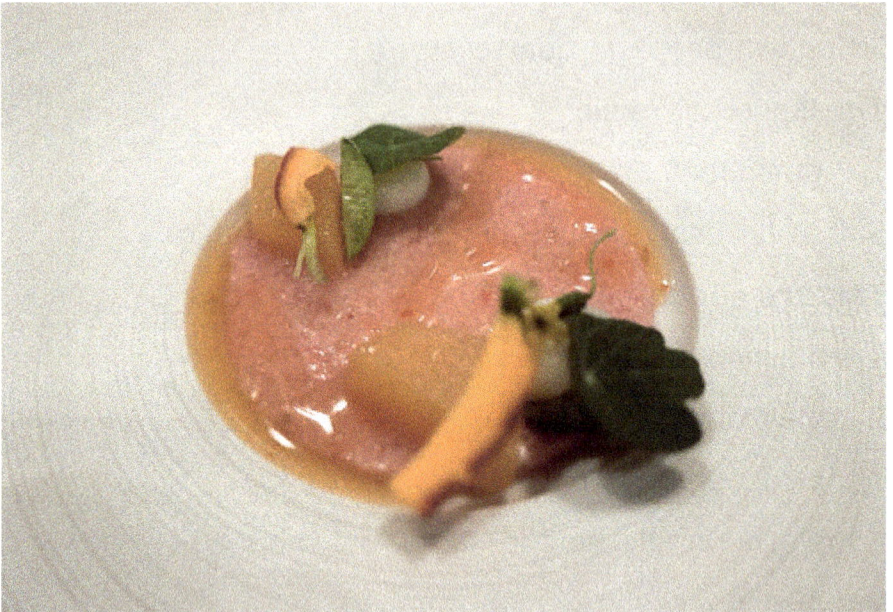

Salmon Filets with Fennel Slaw

Cook Time:

15 minutes

Serving:3

Ingredients:

1 pound salmon filets

1 teaspoon Cajun spice mix

Sea salt and ground black pepper, to taste

Fennel Slaw:

1 pound fennel bulb, thinly sliced

1 Lebanese cucumber, thinly sliced

1/2 red onion, thinly sliced

1/2 ounce tarragon

2 tablespoons tahini

2 tablespoons lemon juice

1 tablespoon soy sauce

Directions:

1.Rinse the salmon filets and pat them dry with a paper towel.

2.Then, toss the salmon filets with the Cajun spice mix, salt and black pepper.

3.Cook the salmon filets in the preheated Air Fryer at 380 degrees F for 6 minutes; flip the salmon filets and cook for a further 6 minutes.

4.Meanwhile, make the fennel slaw by stirring fennel, cucumber, red onion and tarragon in a salad bowl. Mix the remaining ingredients to make the dressing.

5.Dress the salad and transfer to your refrigerator until ready to serve. Serve the warm fish with chilled fennel slaw. Enjoy!

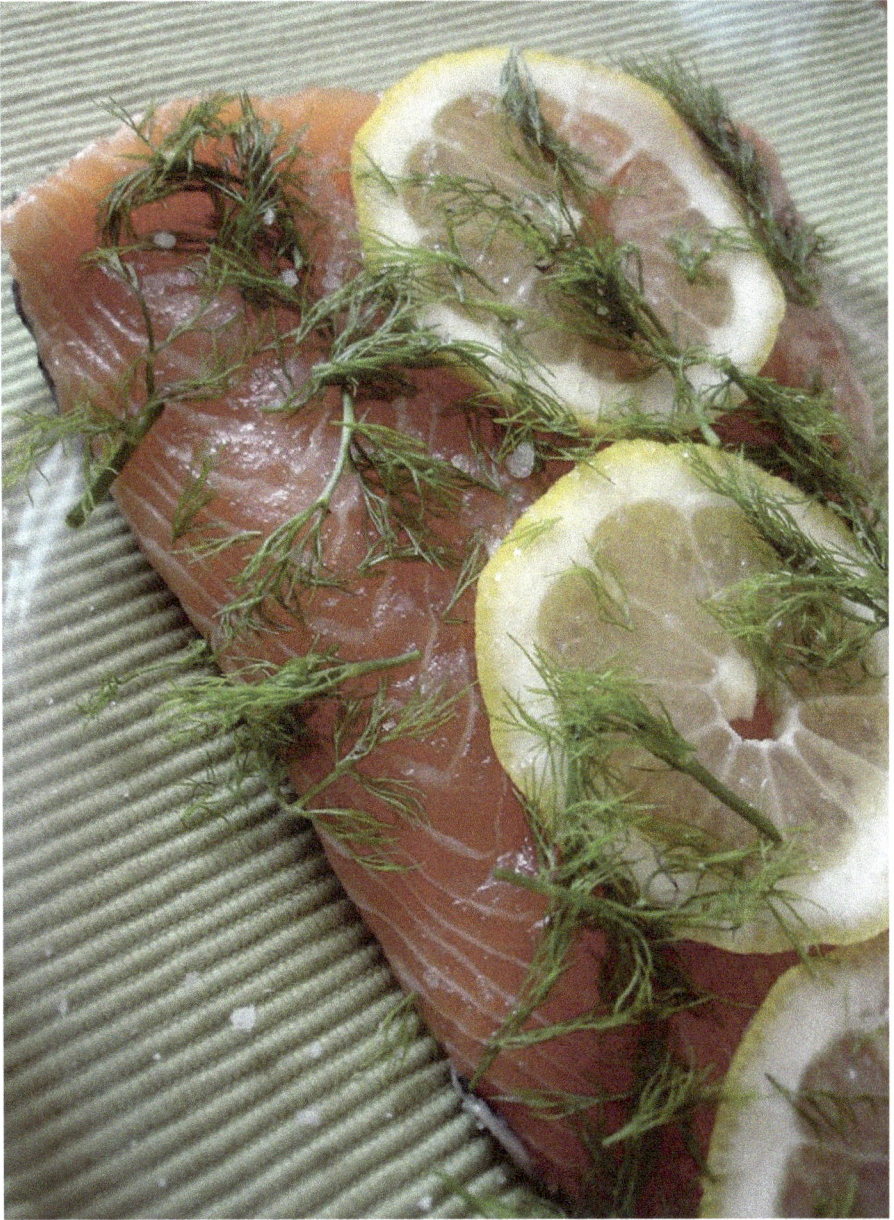

Tortilla-Crusted Haddock Fillets

Cook Time:

20 minutes

Servings:2

Ingredients:

2 haddock fillets

1/2 cup tortilla chips, crushed

2 tablespoons parmesan cheese, freshly grated

1 teaspoon dried parsley flakes

1 egg, beaten

1/2 teaspoon coarse sea salt

1/4 teaspoon ground black pepper

1/4 teaspoon cayenne pepper

2 tablespoons olive oil

Directions:

1.Start by preheating your Air Fryer to 360 degrees F. Pat dry the haddock fillets and set aside.

2.In a shallow bowl, thoroughly combine the crushed tortilla chips with the parmesan and parsley flakes. Mix until everything is well incorporated.

3.In a separate shallow bowl, whisk the egg with salt, black pepper, and cayenne pepper. Dip the haddock fillets into the egg.

4. Then, dip the fillets into the tortilla/parmesan mixture until well coated on all sides.

5. Drizzle the olive oil all over the fish fillets. Lower the coated fillets into the lightly greased Air Fryer basket. Cook for 11 to 13 minutes. Serve and enjoy!

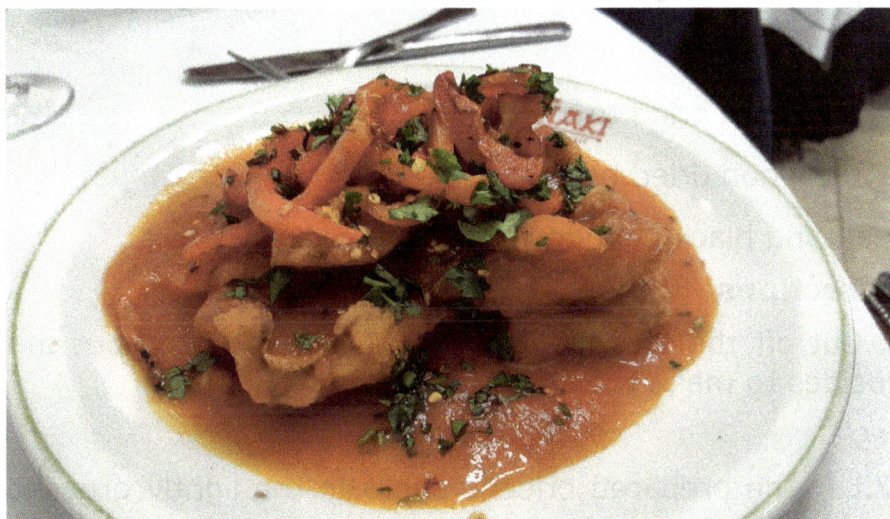

Smoked Halibut and Eggs in Brioche

Cook Time:

25 minutes

Servings:4

Ingredients:

4 brioche rolls

1 pound smoked halibut, chopped

4 eggs

1 teaspoon dried thyme

1 teaspoon dried basil

Salt and black pepper, to taste

Directions:

1.Cut off the top of each brioche; then, scoop out the insides to make the shells.

2.Lay the prepared brioche shells in the lightly greased cooking basket.

3.Spritz with cooking oil; add the halibut. Crack an egg into each brioche shell; sprinkle with thyme, basil, salt, and black pepper.

4.Bake in the preheated Air Fryer at 325 degrees F for 20 minutes. Serve and enjoy!

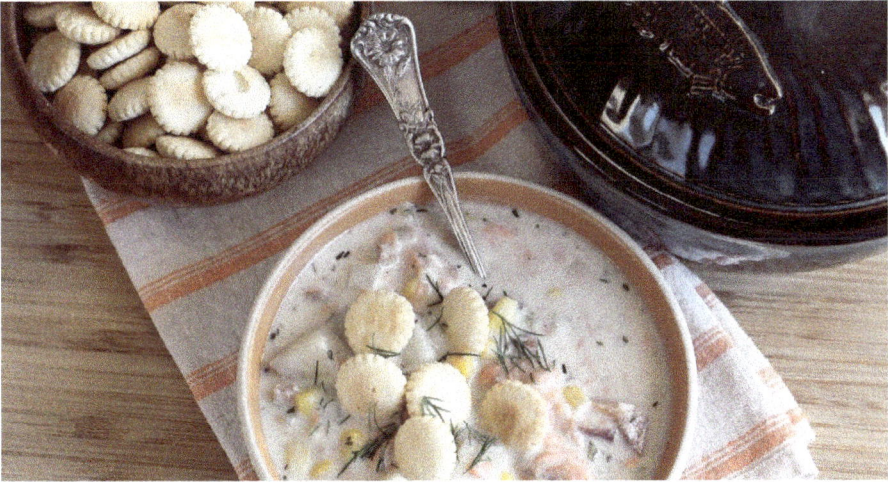

Monkfish Fillets with Romano Cheese

Cook Time:

15 minutes

Servings:2

Ingredients:

2 monkfish fillets

1 teaspoon garlic paste

2 tablespoons butter, melted

1/2 teaspoon Aleppo chili powder

1/2 teaspoon dried rosemary

1/4 teaspoon cracked black pepper

1/2 teaspoon sea salt

4 tablespoons Romano cheese, grated

Directions:

1.Start by preheating the Air Fryer to 320 degrees F. Spritz the Air Fryer basket with cooking oil.

2.Spread the garlic paste all over the fish fillets. Brush the monkfish fillets with the melted butter on both sides.

3.Sprinkle with the chili powder, rosemary, black pepper, and salt.

4.Cook for 7 minutes in the preheated Air Fryer. Top with the Romano cheese and continue to cook for 2 minutes more or until heated through. Serve and enjoy!

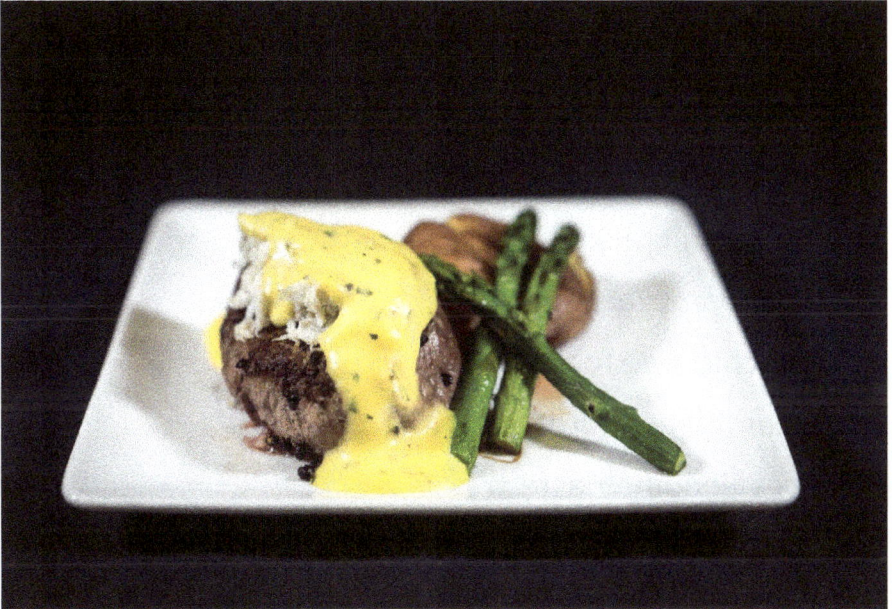

Shrimp Scampi Linguine

Cook Time:

25 minutes

Servings:4

Ingredients:

1 ½ pounds shrimp, shelled and deveined

1/2 tablespoon fresh basil leaves, chopped

2 tablespoons olive oil

2 cloves garlic, minced

1/2 teaspoon fresh ginger, grated

1/4 teaspoon cracked black pepper

1/2 teaspoon sea salt

1/4 cup chicken stock

2 ripe tomatoes, pureed

8 ounces linguine pasta

1/2 cup parmesan cheese, preferably freshly grated

Directions:

1.Start by preheating the Air Fryer to 395 degrees F. Place the shrimp, basil, olive oil, garlic, ginger, black pepper, salt, chicken stock, and tomatoes in the casserole dish.

2.Transfer the casserole dish to the cooking basket and bake for 10 minutes. Bring a large pot of lightly salted water to a boil.

3.Cook the linguine for 10 minutes or until al dente; drain. Divide between four serving plates. Add the shrimp sauce and top with parmesan cheese. Enjoy!

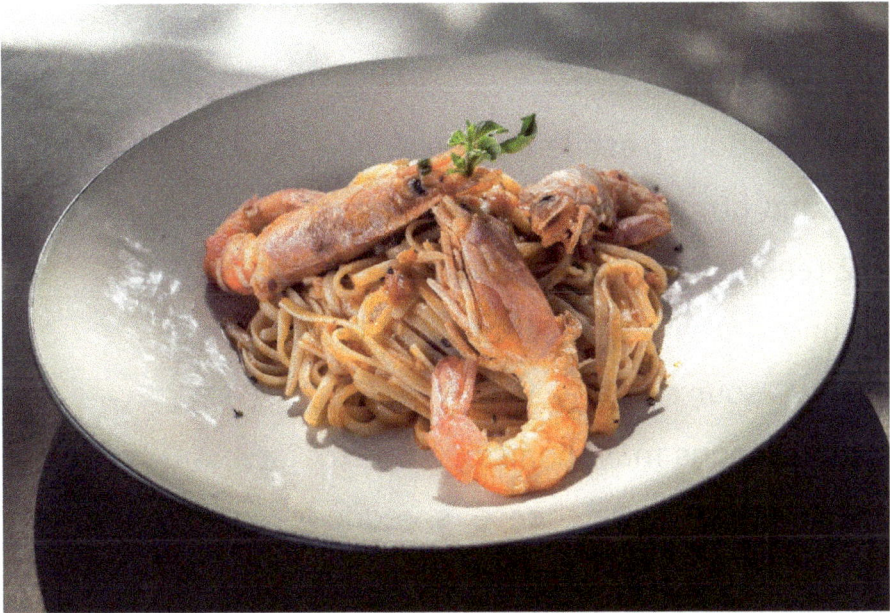

Shrimp Scampi Dip with Cheese

Cook Time:

25 minutes

Servings:8

Ingredients:

2 teaspoons butter, melted

8 ounces shrimp, peeled and deveined

2 garlic cloves, minced

1/4 cup chicken stock

2 tablespoons fresh lemon juice

Salt and ground black pepper, to taste

1/2 teaspoon red pepper flakes

4 ounces cream cheese, at room temperature

1/2 cup sour cream

4 tablespoons mayonnaise

1/4 cup mozzarella cheese, shredded

Directions:

1.Start by preheating the Air Fryer to 395 degrees F. Grease the sides and bottom of a baking dish with the melted butter.

2.Place the shrimp, garlic, chicken stock, lemon juice, salt, black pepper, and red pepper flakes in the baking dish.

3.Transfer the baking dish to the cooking basket and bake for 10 minutes.

4.Add the mixture to your food processor; pulse until the coarsely is chopped.

5.Add the cream cheese, sour cream, and mayonnaise.

6.Top with the mozzarella cheese and bake in the preheated Air Fryer at 360 degrees F for 6 to 7 minutes or until the cheese is bubbling.

7.Serve immediately with breadsticks if desired.

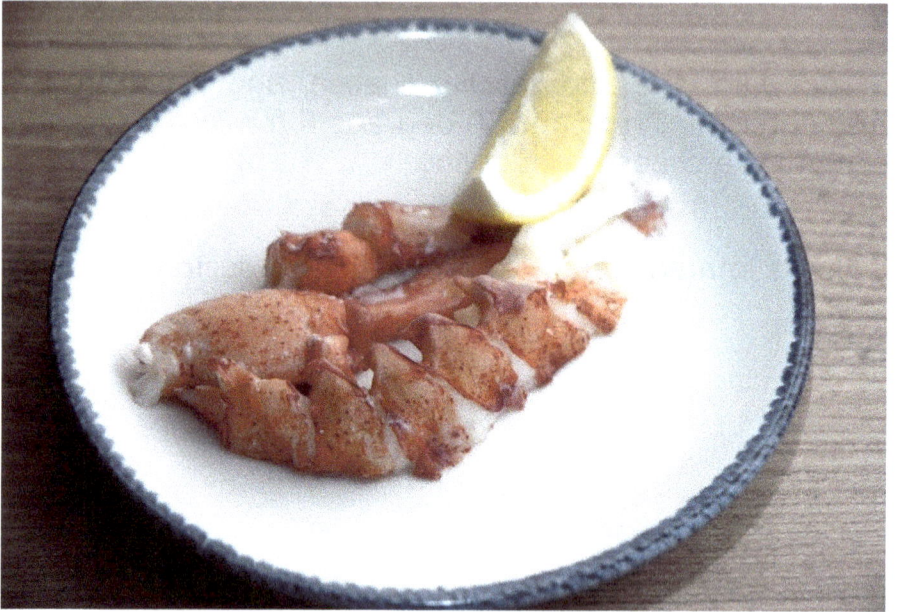

Creamed Trout Salad

Cook Time:

20 minutes

Servings:2

Ingredients:

1/2 pound trout fillets skinless

2 tablespoons horseradish, prepared, drained

1/4 cup mayonnaise

1 tablespoon fresh lemon juice

1 teaspoon mustard

Salt and ground white pepper, to taste

6 ounces chickpeas, canned and drained

1 red onion, thinly sliced

1 cup Iceberg lettuce, torn into pieces

Directions:

1.Spritz the Air Fryer basket with cooking spray. Cook the trout fillets in the preheated Air Fryer at 395 degrees F for 10 minutes or until opaque.

2.Make sure to turn them halfway through the cooking time.

3.Break the fish into bite-sized chunks and place in the refrigerator to cool. Toss your fish with the remaining ingredients. Serve and enjoy!

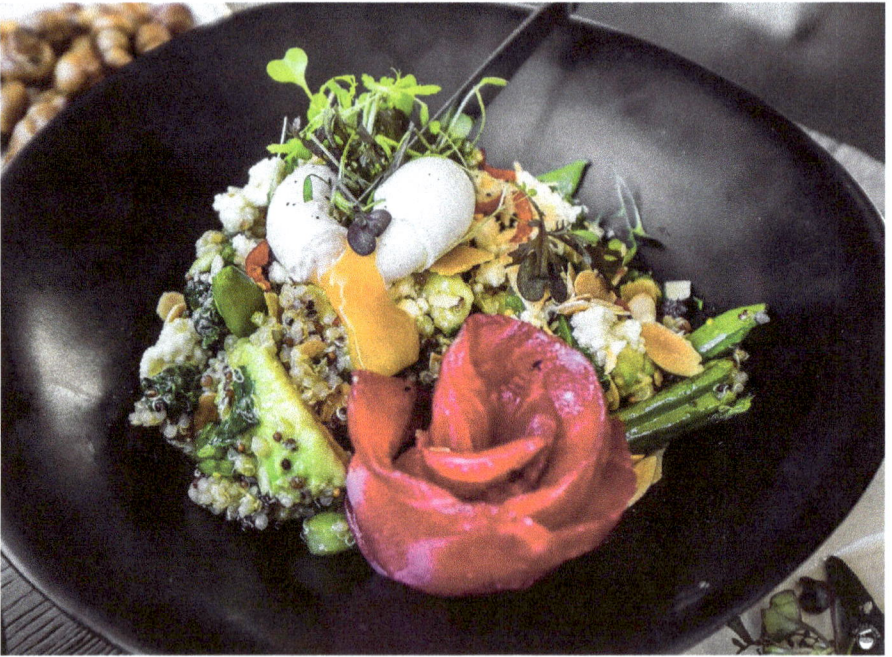

Double Cheese Fish Casserole

Cook Time:

30 minutes.

Servings:4

Ingredients:

1 tablespoon avocado oil

1 pound hake fillets

1 teaspoon garlic powder

Sea salt and ground white pepper, to taste

2 tablespoons shallots, chopped

1 bell pepper, seeded and chopped

1/2 cup Cottage cheese

1/2 cup sour cream

1 egg, well whisked

1 teaspoon yellow mustard

1 tablespoon lime juice

1/2 cup Swiss cheese, shredded

Directions:

1.Brush the bottom and sides of a casserole dish with avocado oil.

2.Add the hake fillets to the casserole dish and sprinkle with garlic powder, salt, and pepper. Add the chopped shallots and bell peppers.

3.In a mixing bowl, thoroughly combine the Cottage cheese, sour cream, egg, mustard, and lime juice.

4.Pour the mixture over fish and spread evenly. Cook in the preheated Air Fryer at 370 degrees F for 10 minutes. Top with the Swiss cheese and cook an additional 7 minutes.

5.Let it rest for 10 minutes before slicing and serving. Enjoy!

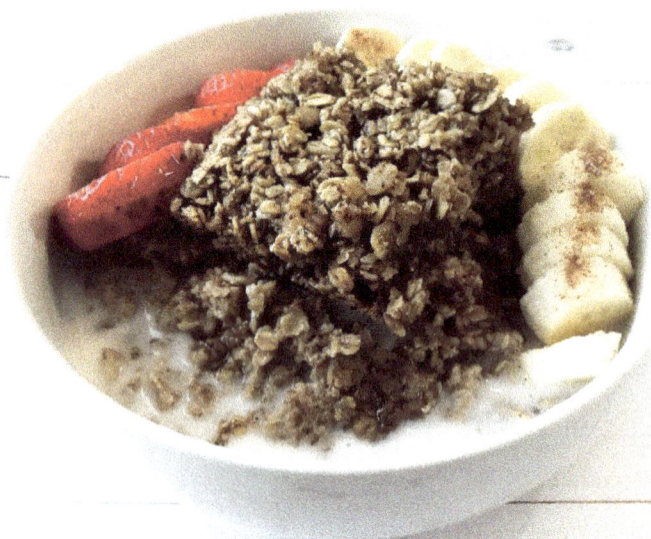

Italian-Style Crab Bruschetta

Cook Time:

15 minutes

Servings:2

Ingredients:

4 slices sourdough bread

2 tablespoons tomato ketchup

4 tablespoons mayonnaise

1 teaspoon fresh rosemary, chopped

8 ounces lump crabmeat

1 teaspoon granulated garlic

2 tablespoons shallots, chopped

4 tablespoons mozzarella cheese, crumbled

Directions:

1.Place the slices of sourdough bread on a flat surface. In a mixing bowl, thoroughly combine the tomato ketchup, mayo, rosemary, crabmeat, garlic, and shallots.

2.Divide the crabmeat mixture between the slices of bread. Top with mozzarella cheese. Bake in the preheated Air Fryer at 370 degrees F for 10 minutes.

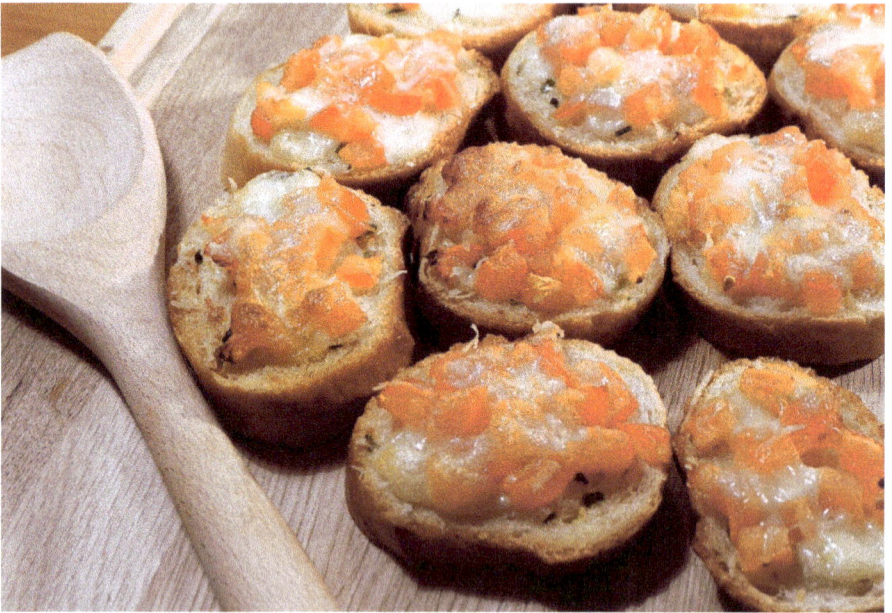

Thai-Style Jumbo Scallops

Cook Time:

40 minutes

Servings: 2

Ingredients:

8 jumbo scallops

1 teaspoon sesame oil

Sea salt and red pepper flakes, to season

1 tablespoon coconut oil

1 Thai chili, deveined and minced

1 teaspoon garlic, minced

1 tablespoon oyster sauce

1 tablespoon soy sauce

1/4 cup coconut milk

2 tablespoons fresh lime juice

Directions:

1.Pat the jumbo scallops dry and toss them with 1 teaspoon of sesame oil, salt and red pepper.

2.Cook the jumbo scallops in your Air Fryer at 400 degrees F for 4 minutes; turn them over and cook an additional 3 minutes.

3.While your scallops are cooking, make the sauce in a frying pan. Heat the coconut oil in a pan over medium-high heat.

4.Once hot, cook the Thai chili and garlic for 1 minute or so until just tender and fragrant.

5.Add in the oyster sauce, soy sauce and coconut milk and continue to simmer, partially covered, for 5 minutes longer.

6.Lastly, stir in fresh lime juice and stir to combine well. Add the warm scallops to the sauce and serve immediately.

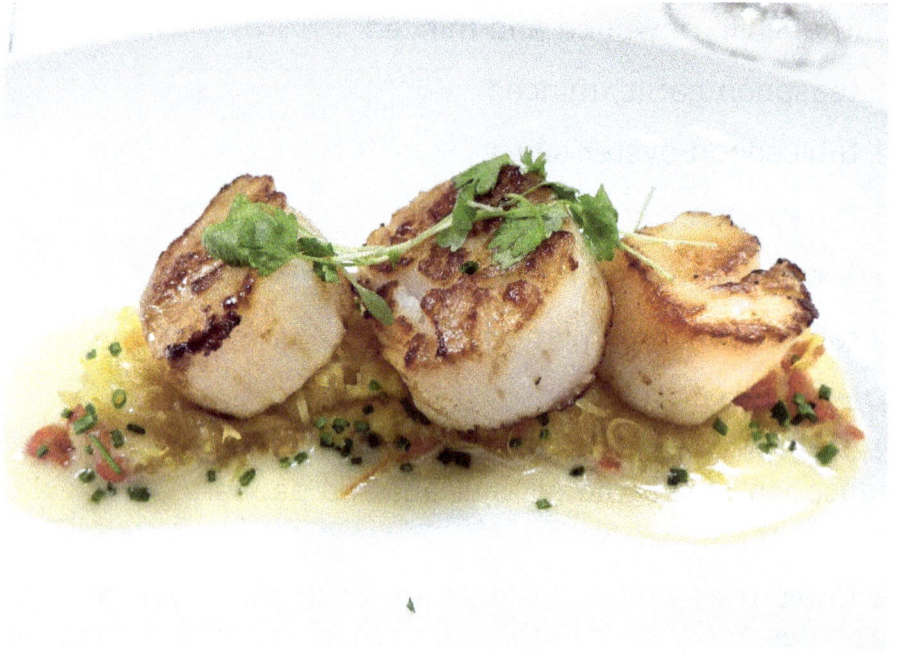

Marinated Flounder Filets

Cook Time:

15 minutes

Servings:3

Ingredients:

1 pound flounder filets

1 teaspoon garlic, minced

2 tablespoons soy sauce

1 teaspoon Dijon mustard

1/4 cup malt vinegar

1 teaspoon granulated sugar

Salt and black pepper, to taste

1/2 cup plain flour

1 egg

2 tablespoons milk

1/2 cup parmesan cheese, grated

Directions:

1.Place the flounder filets, garlic, soy sauce, mustard, vinegar and sugar in a glass bowl; cover and let it marinate in your refrigerator for at least 1 hour.

2.Transfer the fish to a plate, discarding the marinade. Salt and pepper to taste.

3.Place the plain flour in a shallow bowl; in another bowl, beat the egg and milk until pale and well combined; add parmesan cheese to the third bowl.

4.Dip the flounder filets in the flour, then in the egg mixture; repeat the process and coat them with the parmesan cheese, pressing to adhere.

5.Cook the flounder filets in the preheated Air Fryer at 400 degrees F for 5 minutes; turn the flounder filets over and cook on the other side for 5 minutes more. Enjoy!

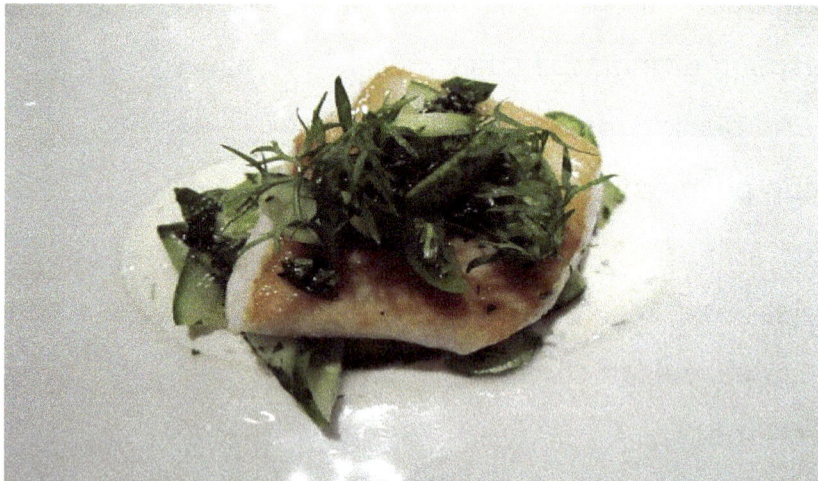

Greek-Style Sea Bass

Cook Time:

15 minutes

Servings:2

Ingredients:

1/2 pound sea bass

1 garlic clove, halved

Sea salt and ground black pepper, to taste

1/2 teaspoon rigani Greek oregano

1/2 teaspoon dried dill weed

1/4 teaspoon ground bay leaf

1/4 teaspoon ground cumin

1/2 teaspoon shallot powder

Greek sauce:

1/2 Greek yogurt

1 teaspoon olive oil

1/2 teaspoon Tzatziki spice mix

1 teaspoon lime juice

Directions:

1.Pat dry the sea bass with paper towels. Rub the fish with garlic halves.

2.Toss the fish with salt, black pepper, rigani, dill, ground bay leaf, ground cumin and shallot powder.

3.Cook the sea bass in your Air Fryer at 400 degrees F for 5 minutes; turn the filets over and cook on the other side for 5 to 6 minutes.

4.In the meantime, make the sauce by simply blending the remaining ingredients. Serve the warm fish dolloped with Greek-style sauce. Enjoy!

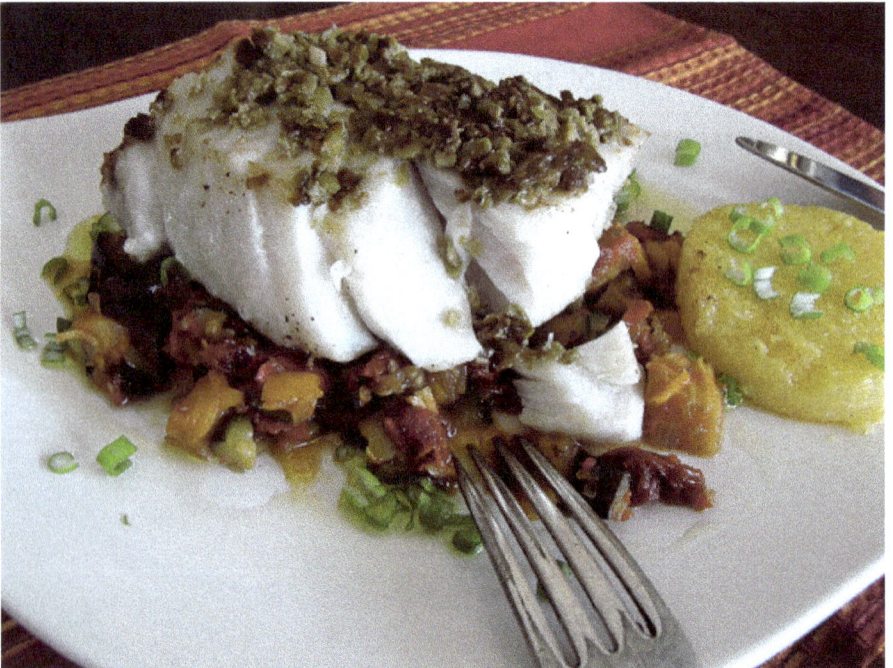

Classic Fish Tacos

Cook Time:

15 minutes

Servings:3

Ingredients:

1 pound codfish

1 tablespoon olive oil

1 teaspoon Cajun spice mix

Salt and red pepper, to taste

3 corn tortillas

1/2 avocado, pitted and diced

1 cup purple cabbage

1 jalapeño, minced

Directions;

1.Pat the codfish dry with paper towels; toss the codfish with olive oil, Cajun spice mix, salt and black pepper. Cook your codfish at 400 degrees F for 5 to 6 minutes.

2.Then, turn the fish over and cook on the other side for 6 minutes until they are opaque.

3.Let the fish rest for 5 minutes before flaking with a fork. Assemble the tacos: place the flaked fish over warmed tortillas; top with avocado, purple cabbage and minced jalapeño. Enjoy!

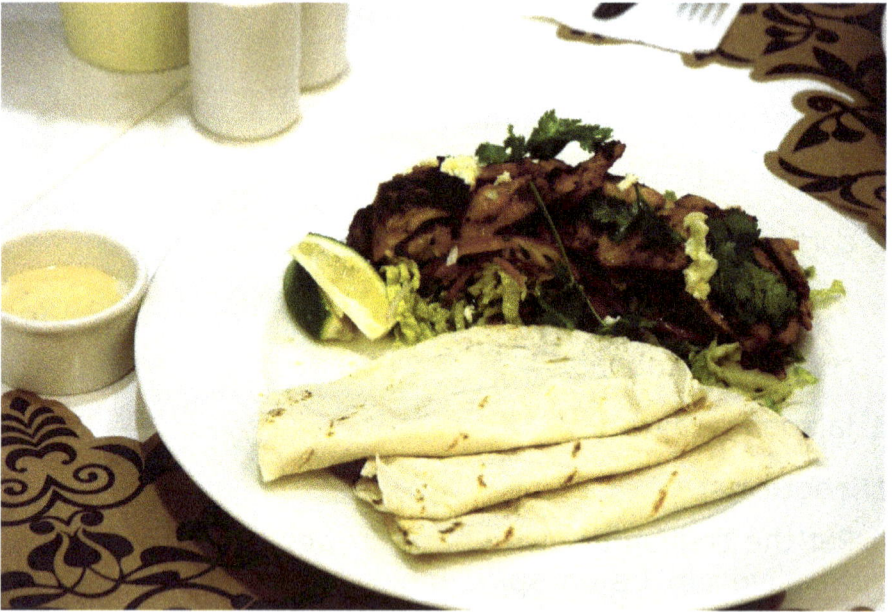

Easy Lobster Tails

Cook Time:

20 minutes

Servings:3

Ingredients:

2 pounds fresh lobster tails, cleaned and halved, in shells
2 tablespoons butter, melted

1 teaspoon onion powder

1 teaspoon cayenne pepper

Salt and ground black pepper, to taste

2 garlic cloves, minced

1 cup cornmeal

1 cup green olives

Directions:

1.In a plastic closeable bag, thoroughly combine all ingredients; shake to combine well.

2.Transfer the coated lobster tails to the greased cooking basket.

3.Cook in the preheated Air Fryer at 390 degrees for 6 to 7 minutes, shaking the basket halfway through. Work in batches. Serve with green olives and enjoy!

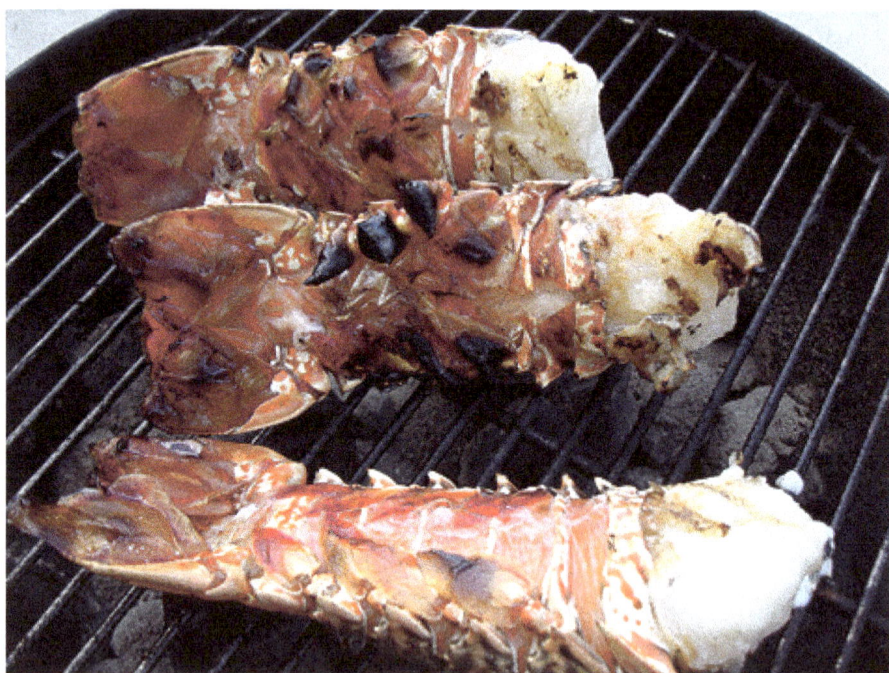

Crunchy Fish Sticks

Preparation Time:

10 minutes

Cooking Time:

15 minutes

Serve: 5

Ingredients:

12 oz tilapia loins, cut into fish sticks

1/2 cup parmesan cheese, grated

3.25 oz pork rind, crushed

1 tsp paprika

1 tsp garlic powder

1/4 cup mayonnaise

Directions:

1.In a shallow bowl, mix together parmesan cheese, crushed pork rind, paprika, and garlic powder.

2.Add fish pieces and mayonnaise into the mixing bowl and mix well.

3.Place the cooking tray in the air fryer basket. Select Air Fry mode. Set time to 15 minutes and temperature 380 F then press START.

4.The air fryer display will prompt you to ADD FOOD once the temperature is reached then coat fish pieces with parmesan mixture and place in the air fryer basket. Serve and enjoy

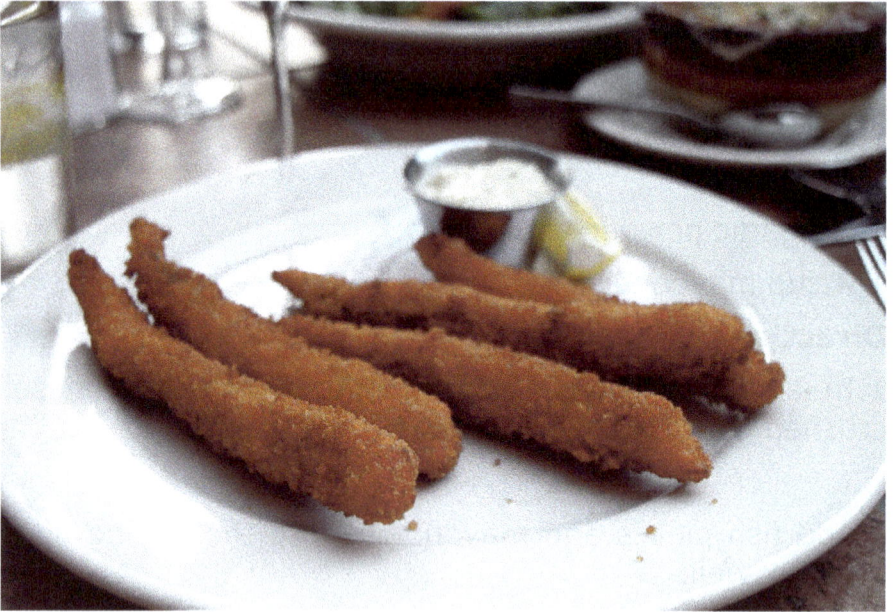

Parmesan Shrimp

Preparation Time:

10 minutes

Cooking Time:

12 minutes

Serve: 4

Ingredients:

1 lb shrimp, peeled & deveined

2 tbsp parsley, minced

2 tbsp parmesan cheese, grated

1/8 tsp garlic powder

2 tbsp olive oil

1/2 tsp pepper

1/2 tsp salt

Directions:

1.In a mixing bowl, toss shrimp with olive oil. Add remaining ingredients and toss until shrimp is well coated. Place the cooking tray in the air fryer basket.

2.Select Air Fry mode. Set time to 12 minutes and temperature 400 F then press START.

3.The air fryer display will prompt you to ADD FOOD once the temperature is reached then add shrimp in the air fryer basket. Stir shrimp halfway through. Serve and enjoy.

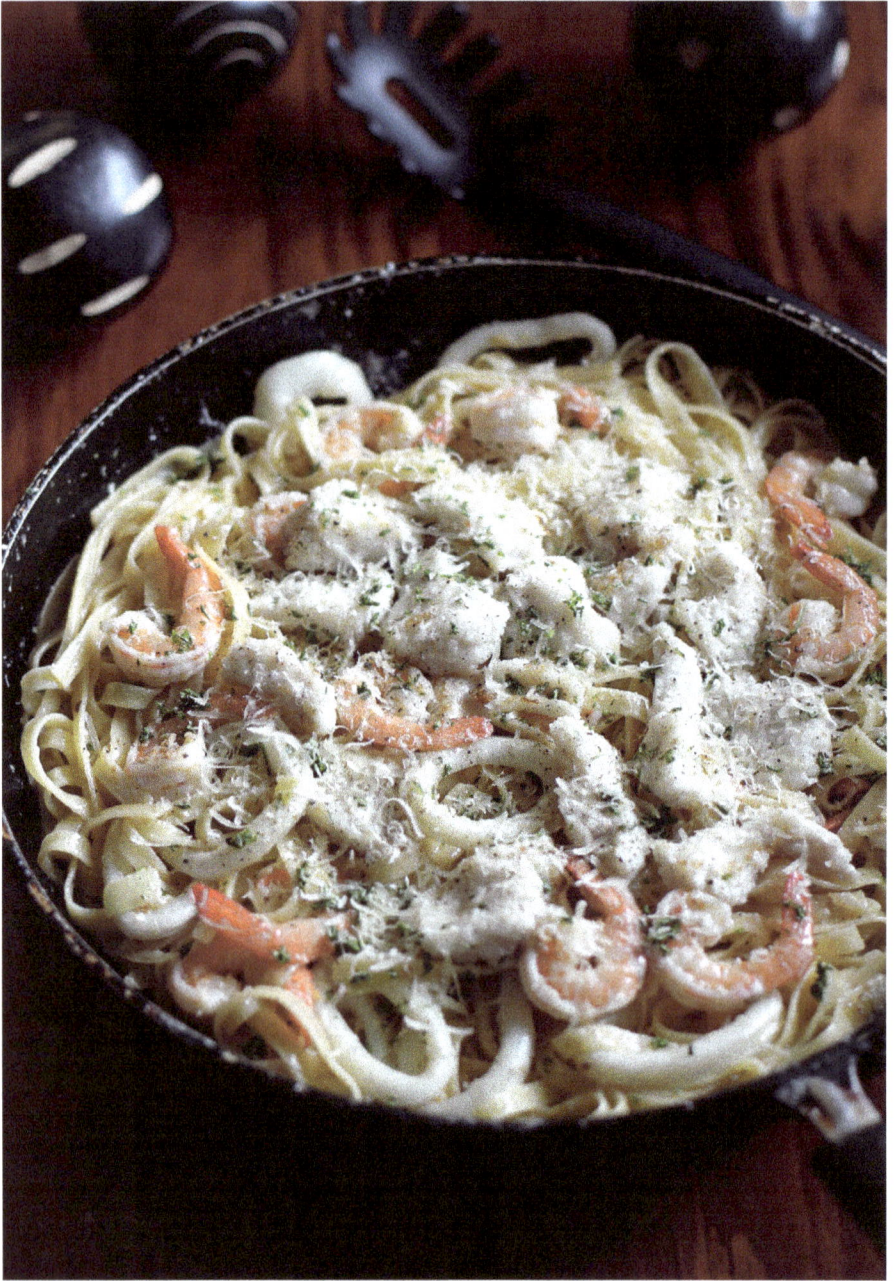

Baked Tilapia

Preparation Time:

10 minutes

Cooking Time:

15 minutes

Serve: 6

Ingredients:

6 tilapia fillets

1/2 cup Asiago cheese, grated

1/4 tsp basil

1/4 tsp thyme

1/4 tsp onion powder

1 tsp garlic, minced

1/2 cup mayonnaise

1/8 tsp pepper

1/4 tsp salt

Directions:

1.In a small bowl, mix together the grated cheese, basil, thyme, onion powder, garlic, mayonnaise, pepper, and salt. Place the cooking tray in the air fryer basket.

2.Line air fryer basket with parchment paper. Select Bake mode. Set time to 15 minutes and temperature 350 F then press START.

3.The air fryer display will prompt you to ADD FOOD once the temperature is reached then place fish fillets in the air fryer basket and spread cheese mixture on top of each fish fillet. Serve and enjoy.

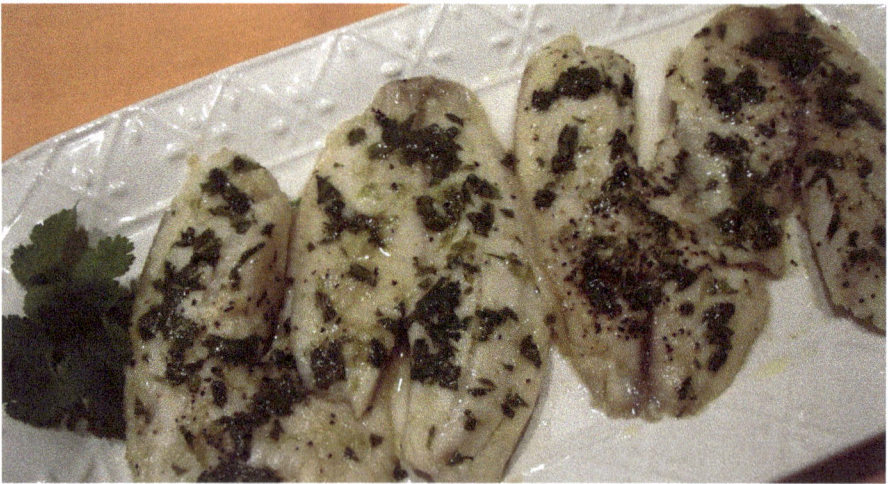

Pecan Crusted Fish Fillets

Preparation Time:

10 minutes

Cooking Time:

17 minutes

Serve: 2

Ingredients:

2 halibut fillets

1/2 lemon juice

1 tsp garlic, minced

1/4 cup parmesan cheese, grated

1/4 cup pecans

2 tbsp butter Pepper Salt

Directions:

1.Add pecans, lemon juice, garlic, parmesan cheese, and butter into the food processor and process until completely blended.

2.Place the cooking tray in the air fryer basket. Line air fryer basket with parchment paper.

3.Select Bake mode. Set time to 5 minutes and temperature 400 F then press START.

4.The air fryer display will prompt you to ADD FOOD once the temperature is reached then season fish fillets with pepper and salt and place in the air fryer basket.

5.Spread pecan mixture on top of fish fillets and bake for 12 minutes more. Serve and enjoy.

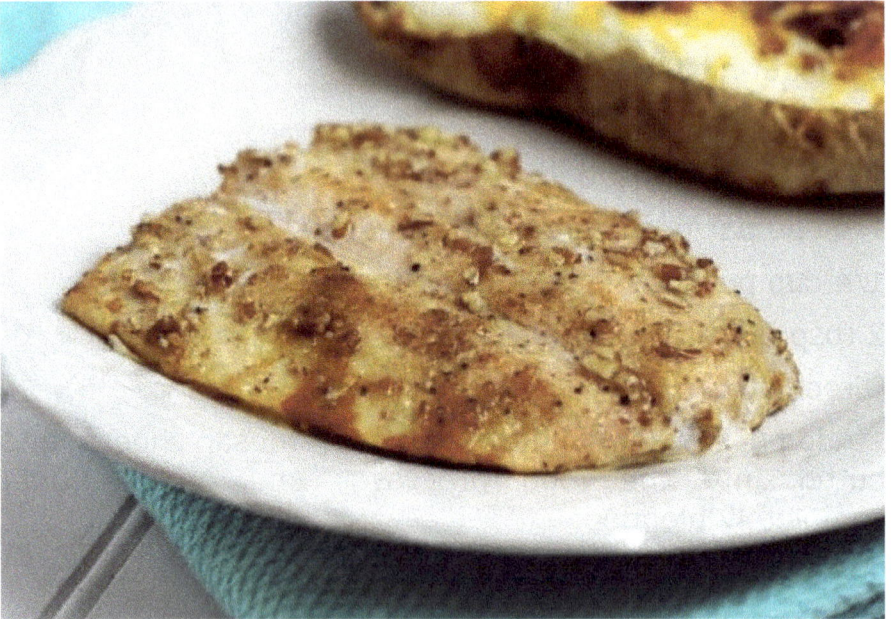

Moist & Juicy Baked Cod

Preparation Time:

10 minutes

Cooking Time:

10 minutes

Serve: 2

Ingredients:

1 lb cod fillets

1 1/2 tbsp olive oil

3 dashes cayenne pepper

1 tbsp lemon juice

1/4 tsp salt

Directions:

1.In a small bowl, mix together olive oil, cayenne pepper, lemon juice, and salt.

2.Brush fish fillets with oil mixture. Place the cooking tray in the air fryer basket. Line air fryer basket with parchment paper. Select Bake mode.

3.Set time to 10 minutes and temperature 400 F then press START. The air fryer display will prompt you to ADD FOOD once the temperature is reached then place fish fillets in the air fryer basket. Serve and enjoy.

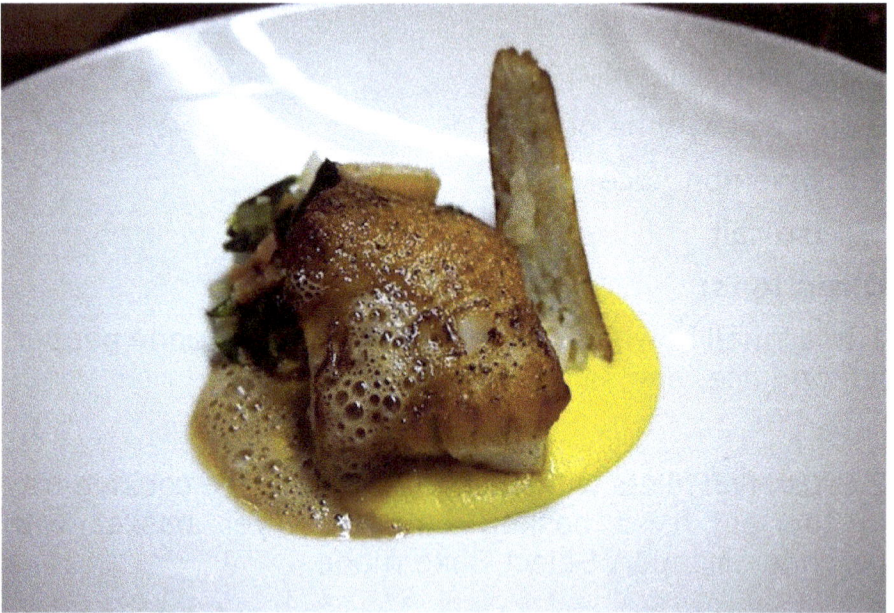

Easy Air Fryer Scallops

Preparation Time:

10 minutes

Cooking Time:

4 minutes

Serve: 2

Ingredients:

8 scallops

1 tbsp olive oil

Pepper Salt

Directions:

1.Brush scallops with olive oil and season with pepper and salt. Place the cooking tray in the air fryer basket. Select Air Fry mode.

2.Set time to 2 minutes and temperature 390 F then press START.

3.The air fryer display will prompt you to ADD FOOD once the temperature is reached then add scallops in the air fryer basket.

4.Turn scallops and air fry for 2 minutes more. Serve and enjoy.

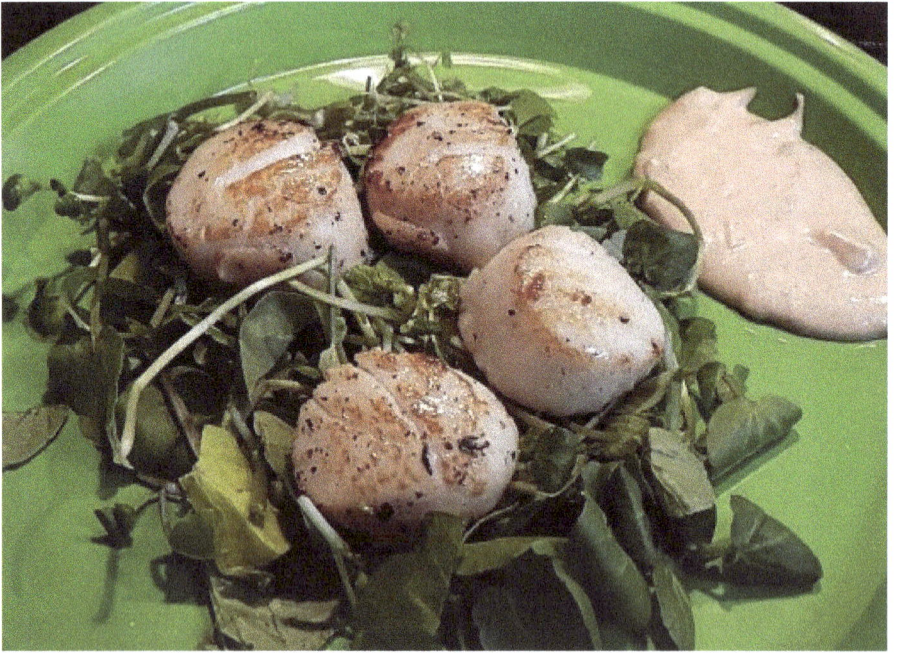

Mayo Cheese Crust Salmon

Preparation Time:

10 minutes

Cooking Time:

14 minutes

Serve: 4

Ingredients:

4 salmon fillets

2 tsp Italian seasoning

2 tbsp parmesan cheese, grated

2 tbsp crushed pork rind

4 tbsp mayonnaise

Directions:

1.Spread mayonnaise on top of fish fillets. Sprinkle with cheese, Italian seasoning, and crushed pork rind.

2.Place the cooking tray in the air fryer basket. Line air fryer basket with parchment paper.

3.Select Bake mode. Set time to 14 minutes and temperature 375 F then press START.

4.The air fryer display will prompt you to ADD FOOD once the temperature is reached then place fish fillets in the air fryer basket. Serve and enjoy.

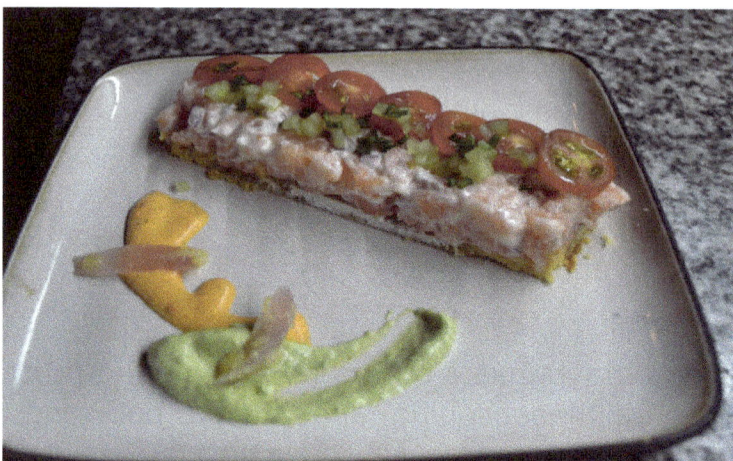

Delicious Crab Cakes

Preparation Time:

10 minutes

Cooking Time:

20 minutes

Serve: 4

Ingredients:

1 lb lump crab meat

1 tbsp butter, melted

1/2 tsp old bay seasoning

1 tbsp parsley, chopped

1 tsp garlic powder

1 tsp onion powder

1/4 cup parmesan cheese

1 egg yolk, lightly beaten

1 egg, lightly beaten

2 tsp Dijon mustard

1/4 cup mayonnaise

Directions:

1.Add all ingredients except melted butter into the mixing bowl and mix until well combined.

2.Make 4 equal shapes of patties from the mixture. Place the cooking tray in the air fryer basket. Line air fryer basket with parchment paper.

3.Select Bake mode. Set time to 20 minutes and temperature 400 F then press START.

4.The air fryer display will prompt you to ADD FOOD once the temperature is reached then place patties in the air fryer basket and drizzle with melted butter. Serve and enjoy.

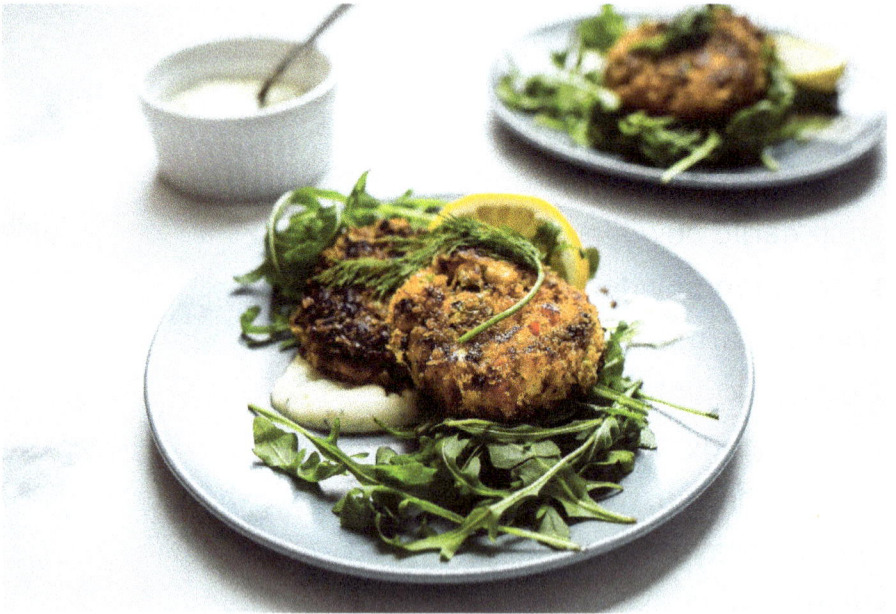

Easy Tuna Patties

Preparation Time:

10 minutes

Cooking Time:

10 minutes

Serve: 5

Ingredients:

15 oz can albacore tuna, drained

1/2 tsp dried mix herbs

1/2 tsp garlic powder

3 tbsp onion, minced

1 celery stalk, chopped

3 tbsp parmesan cheese, grated

1/2 cup almond flour

1 tbsp lemon juice

2 large eggs, lightly beaten

Directions:

1.Add all ingredients into the mixing bowl and mix until well combined.

2.Make the equal shape of patties from the mixture. Place the cooking tray in the air fryer basket. Line air fryer basket with parchment paper.

3.Select Air Fry mode. Set time to 10 minutes and temperature 360 F then press START.

4.The air fryer display will prompt you to ADD FOOD once the temperature is reached then place patties in the air fryer basket. Turn patties halfway through. Serve and enjoy

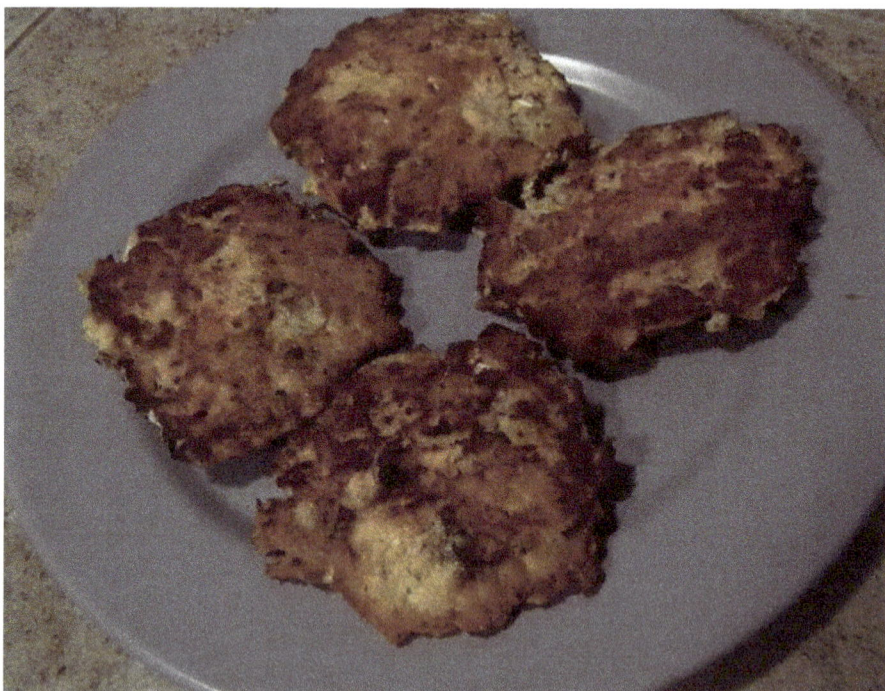

Baked Basa

Preparation Time:

10 minutes

Cooking Time:

30 minutes

Serve: 2

Ingredients:

2 basa fish fillets

4 lemon slices

1/8 tsp lemon juice

1/2 tbsp dried basil

1/2 tsp paprika

4 tsp butter, melted

1/8 tsp salt

Directions:

1.In a small bowl, mix together butter, paprika, basil, lemon juice, and salt. Brush fish fillets with melted butter mixture.

2.Place the cooking tray in the air fryer basket. Line air fryer basket with parchment paper. Select Air Fry mode. Set time to 30 minutes and temperature 350 F then press START.

3.The air fryer display will prompt you to ADD FOOD once the temperature is reached then place fish fillets in the air fryer basket and place lemon slices on fish fillets.

4.Turn fish fillets halfway through. Serve and enjoy.

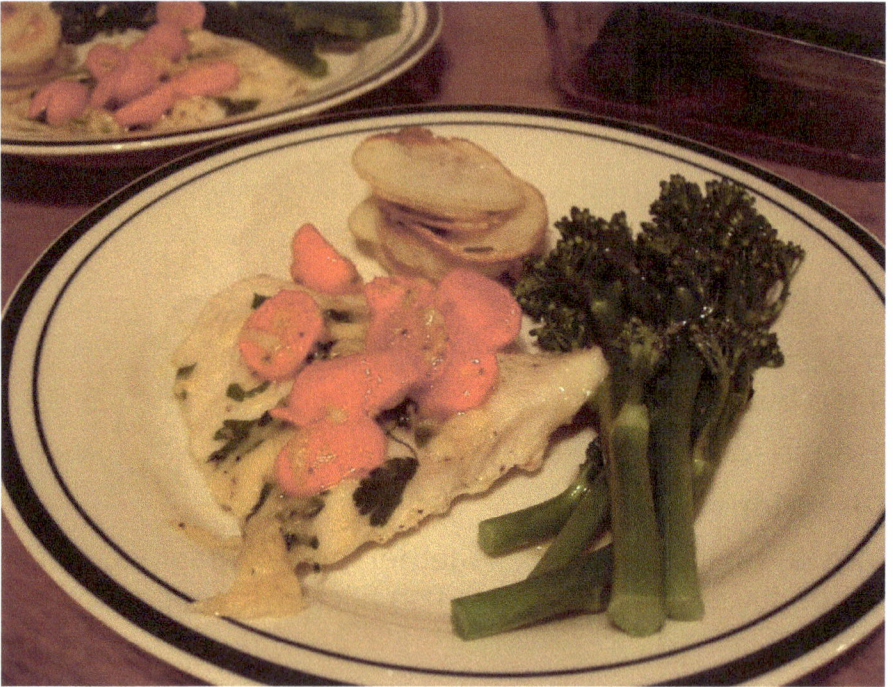

Old Bay Baked Cod

Preparation Time:

10 minutes

Cooking Time:

15 minutes

Serve: 4

Ingredients:

1 lb cod fillets

1/8 tsp dried basil

1/8 tsp old bay seasoning

1 tbsp lemon juice

1 1/2 tbsp mayonnaise

2 tbsp butter, melted

1/4 cup parmesan cheese, grated

Directions:

1.In a bowl, mix together parmesan cheese, butter, mayonnaise, lemon juice, old bay seasoning, and basil. Spread parmesan cheese mixture on top of fish fillets.

2.Place the cooking tray in the air fryer basket. Line air fryer basket with parchment paper. Select Bake mode. Set time to 15 minutes and temperature 350 F then press START.

3.The air fryer display will prompt you to ADD FOOD once the temperature is reached then place the fish fillet in the air fryer basket. Serve and enjoy.

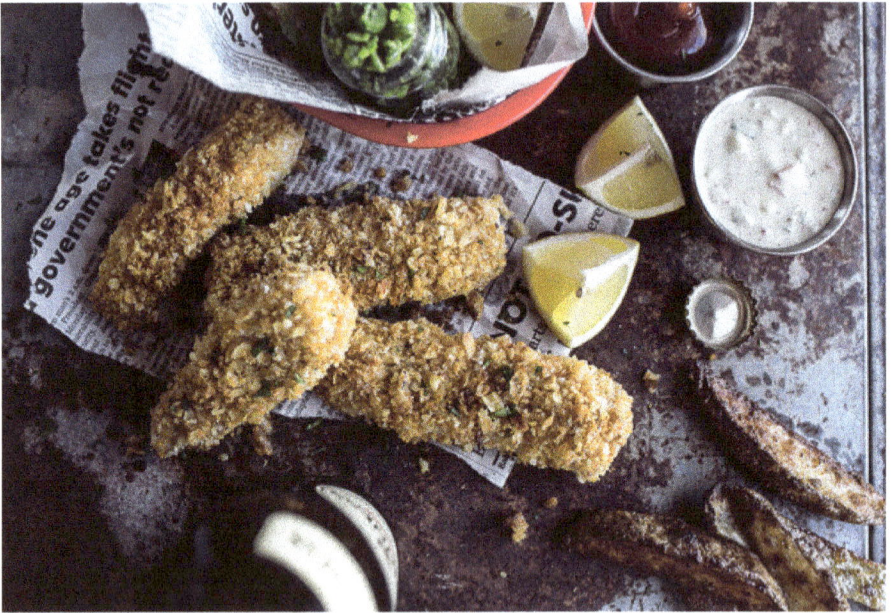

Blackened Tilapia

Preparation Time: 10 minutes

Cooking Time: 14 minutes

Serve: 3

Ingredients:

3 tilapia fillets

1 tbsp dried parsley flakes

1/4 tsp cayenne pepper

1 tsp garlic powder

1 tsp onion powder

2 1/2 tbsp paprika

1/2 tsp pepper

1 tsp salt

Directions:

1.In a small bowl, mix together paprika, pepper, onion powder, garlic powder, cayenne, parsley, pepper, and salt. Spray fish fillets with cooking spray.

2.Rub the paprika mixture on both sides of fish fillets. Place the cooking tray in the air fryer basket. Line air fryer basket with parchment paper.

3.Select Bake mode. Set time to 14 minutes and temperature 400 F then press START.

4.The air fryer display will prompt you to ADD FOOD once the temperature is reached then place the fish fillet in the air fryer basket. Serve and enjoy.

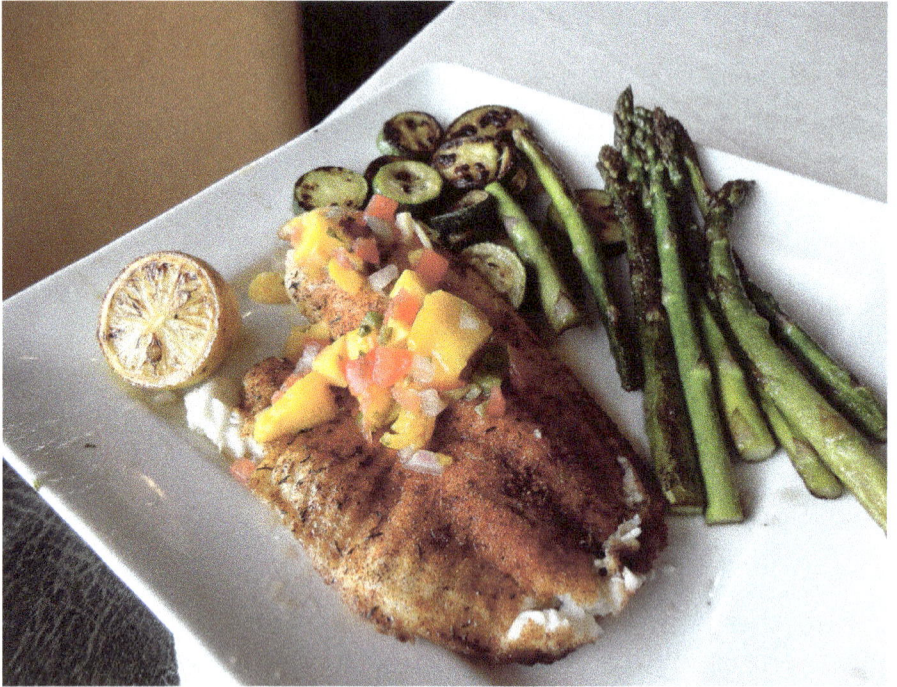

Garlic Butter Baked Shrimp

Preparation Time:

10 minutes

Cooking Time:

8 minutes

Serve: 4

Ingredients:

1 1/2 lbs shrimp, peeled & deveined

1/4 cup parmesan cheese, grated

1/2 tsp paprika

1 tsp garlic powder

1/4 tsp pepper

1/4 cup butter, melted

1 tsp kosher salt

Directions:

1.Add shrimp and remaining ingredients into the large bowl and toss well. Place the cooking tray in the air fryer basket. Line air fryer basket with parchment paper. Select Bake mode.

2.Set time to 8 minutes and temperature 400 F then press START.

3.The air fryer display will prompt you to ADD FOOD once the temperature is reached then add shrimp in the air fryer basket. Serve and enjoy.

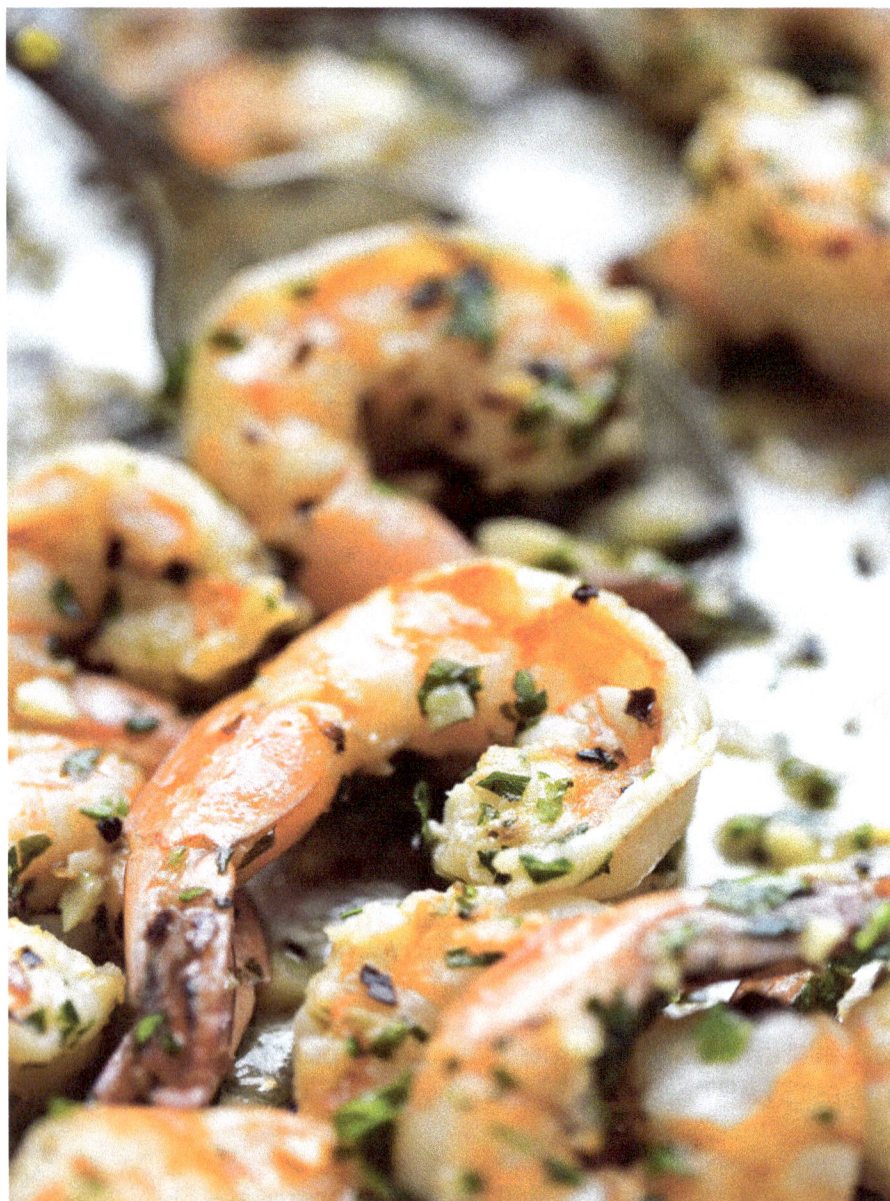

Cajun Catfish Fillets

Preparation Time:

10 minutes

Cooking Time:

25 minutes

Serve: 2

Ingredients:

2 catfish fillets

1/2 tbsp olive oil

1/2 tsp red pepper flakes, crushed

1/2 tsp oregano

1/2 tsp paprika

1/2 tsp cayenne pepper

1/2 tsp onion powder

1/2 tsp garlic powder

Pepper Salt

Directions:

1.In a small bowl, mix together garlic powder, onion powder, cayenne pepper, paprika, oregano, red pepper flakes, pepper, and salt.

2.Brush fish fillets with olive oil and rub with spice mixture. Place the cooking tray in the air fryer basket. Line air fryer basket with parchment paper.

3.Select Bake mode. Set time to 25 minutes and temperature 350 F then press START.

4.The air fryer display will prompt you to ADD FOOD once the temperature is reached then place fish fillets in the air fryer basket. Serve and enjoy.

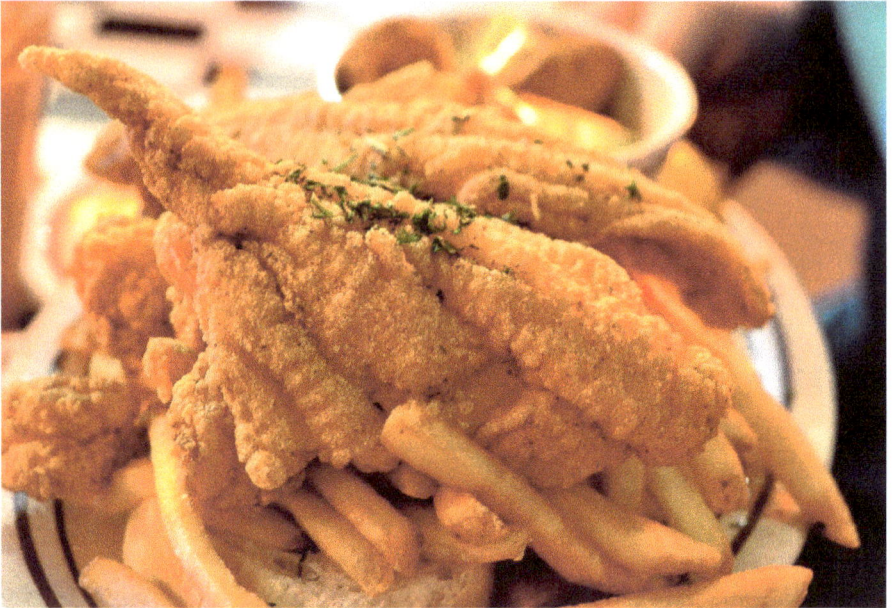

Lemon Garlic Shrimp

Preparation Time:

10 minutes

Cooking Time:

14 minutes

Serve: 3

Ingredients:

1 lb shrimp, peeled & deveined

1/4 tsp garlic powder

1 tbsp olive oil

1/2 lemon

Pepper Salt

Directions:

1.In a mixing bowl, toss shrimp with garlic powder, olive oil, pepper, and salt. Place the cooking tray in the air fryer basket.

2.Select Air Fry mode. Set time to 14 minutes and temperature 400 F then press START.

3.The air fryer display will prompt you to ADD FOOD once the temperature is reached then add shrimp in the air fryer basket. Shake basket halfway through.

4.Squeeze lemon juice over shrimp and serve.

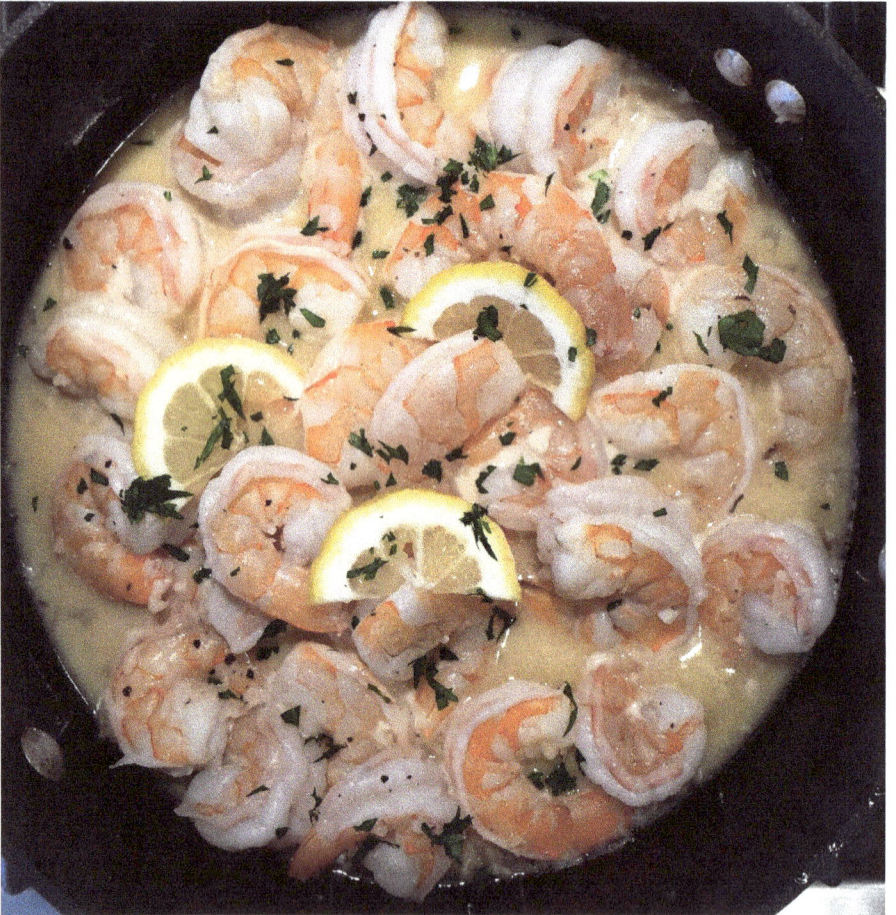

Cod with Vegetables

Preparation Time:

10 minutes

Cooking Time:

15 minutes

Serve: 4

Ingredients:

1 lb cod fillets

1/2 tsp paprika

1/4 cup olive oil

1/4 cup lemon juice 8 oz asparagus, chopped

3 cups broccoli, chopped

1/2 tsp lemon pepper seasoning

1 tsp salt

Directions:

1.In a small bowl, mix together lemon juice, paprika, olive oil, lemon pepper seasoning, and salt. Place the cooking tray in the air fryer basket.

2.Line air fryer basket with parchment paper. Select Bake mode. Set time to 15 minutes and temperature 400 F then press START.

3.The air fryer display will prompt you to ADD FOOD once the temperature is reached.

4.Then place fish fillets in the middle of the parchment paper in the air fryer basket.

5.Place broccoli and asparagus around the fish fillets. Pour lemon juice mixture over the fish fillets. Serve and enjoy.

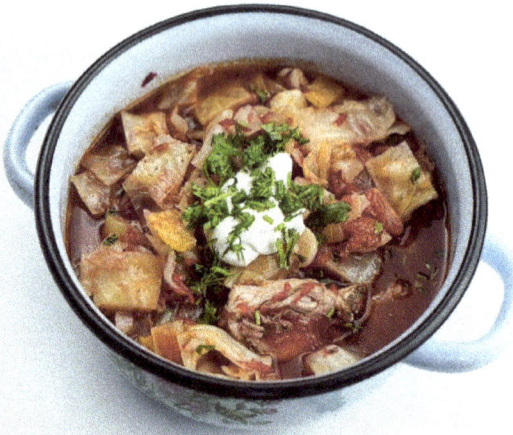

Healthy Swordfish Fillets

Preparation Time:

10 minutes

Cooking Time:

20 minutes

Serve: 2

Ingredients:

12 oz swordfish fillets

1 garlic clove, minced

2 tsp fresh parsley, chopped

3 tbsp olive oil

1/2 tsp lemon zest, grated

1/2 tsp ginger, grated

1/8 tsp crushed red pepper

Directions:

1.In a small bowl, mix together 2 tablespoon oil, lemon zest, red pepper, ginger, garlic, and parsley. Season fish fillets with salt.

2.Heat remaining oil in a pan over medium-high heat. Place fish fillets in the pan and cook until lightly browned 2-3 minutes.

3.Select Bake mode. Set time to 10 minutes and temperature 400 F then press START.

4. The air fryer display will prompt you to ADD FOOD once the temperature is reached then place fish fillets in the air fryer basket. Pour oil mixture over fish fillets and serve.

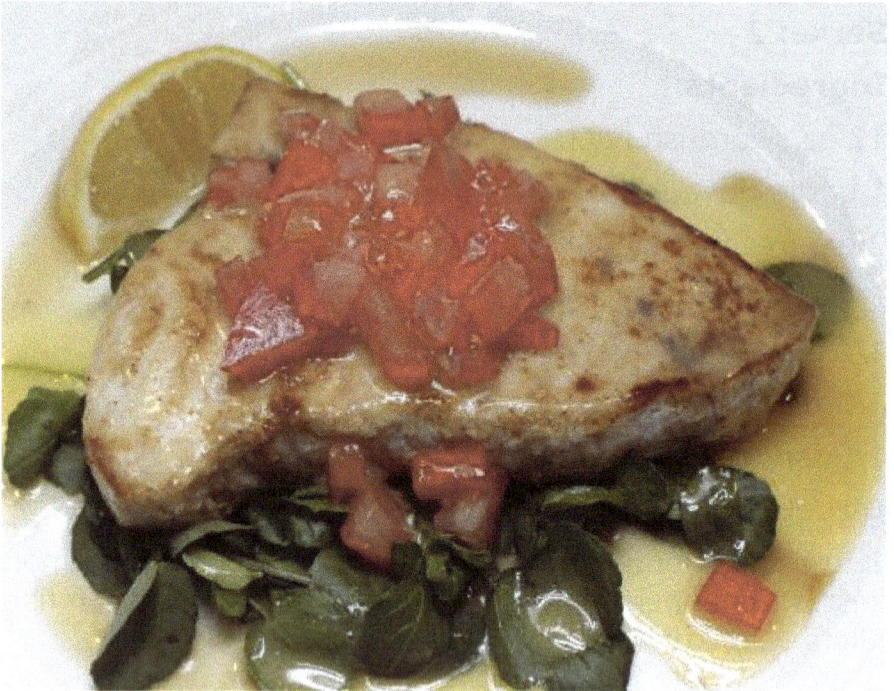

Air Fry Fish Patties

Preparation Time:

10 minutes

Cooking Time:

6 minutes

Serve: 4

Ingredients:

1 egg, lightly beaten

1/4 cup almond flour

8 oz can tuna, drained

1 tbsp mustard

Pepper Salt

Directions:

1.Add all ingredients into the large bowl and mix until well combined. Make four equal shapes of patties from the mixture.

2.Select Air Fry mode. Set time to 6 minutes and temperature 400 F then press START.

3.The air fryer display will prompt you to ADD FOOD once the temperature is reached then place patties in the air fryer basket. Turn patties halfway through. Serve and enjoy.

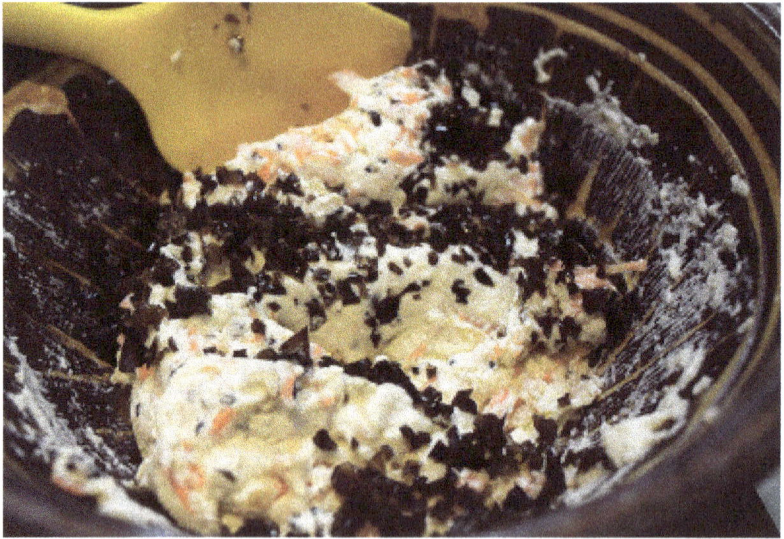

Delicious Shrimp Fajitas

Preparation Time:

10 minutes

Cooking Time:

22 minutes

Serve: 12

Ingredients:

1 lb shrimp

1/2 cup onion, diced

2 bell pepper, diced

1 tbsp olive oil

2 tbsp taco seasoning

Directions:

1.Add shrimp and remaining ingredients into the bowl and toss well.

2.Select Air Fry mode. Set time to 22 minutes and temperature 390 F then press START.

3.The air fryer display will prompt you to ADD FOOD once the temperature is reached then place shrimp mixture in the air fryer basket. Stir halfway through. Serve and enjoy.

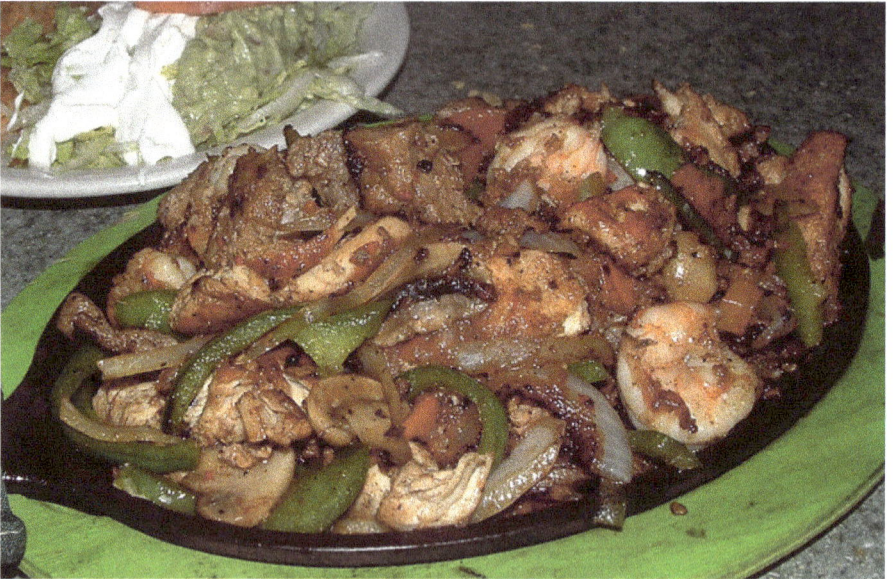

Tasty Crab Patties

Preparation Time:

10 minutes

Cooking Time:

10 minutes

Serve: 4

Ingredients:

8 oz crab meat

2 tbsp mayonnaise

2 green onion, chopped

1/4 cup bell pepper, chopped

1 tsp old bay seasoning

1 tbsp Dijon mustard

2 tbsp almond flour

Pepper Salt

Directions:

1.Add all ingredients into the mixing bowl and mix until well combined. Make 4 equal shapes of patties from the mixture.

2.Select Air Fry mode. Set time to 10 minutes and temperature 370 F then press START.

3.The air fryer display will prompt you to ADD FOOD once the temperature is reached then place patties in the air fryer basket. Serve and enjoy.

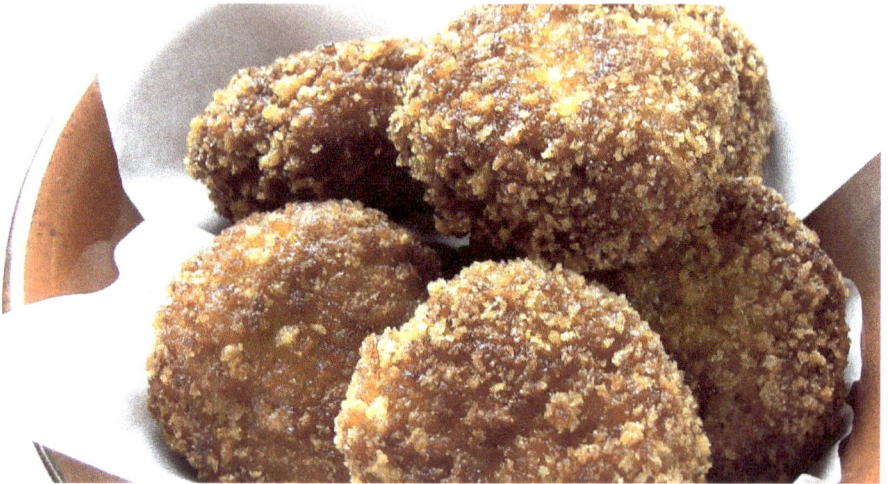

Cajun Scallops

Preparation Time:

10 minutes

Cooking Time:

6 minutes

Serve: 1

Ingredients:

4 scallops, rinsed and pat dry

1/2 tsp Cajun seasoning

Pepper Salt

Directions:

1.Spray scallops with cooking spray and season with Cajun seasoning, pepper, and salt.

2.Select Air Fry mode. Set time to 6 minutes and temperature 400 F then press START.

3.The air fryer display will prompt you to ADD FOOD once the temperature is reached then place scallops in the air fryer basket. Turn scallops halfway through. Serve and enjoy.

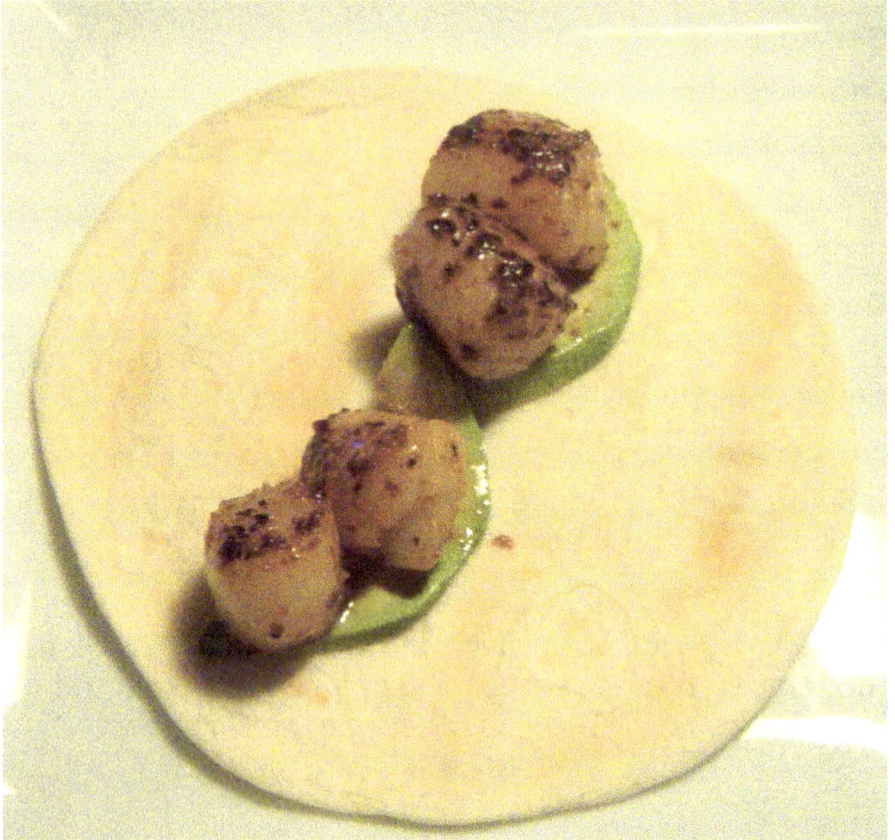

Greek Baked Salmon

Preparation Time:

10 minutes

Cooking Time:

20 minutes

Serve: 5

Ingredients:

1 3/4 lbs salmon fillet

1/3 cup artichoke hearts

1/4 cup sun-dried tomatoes, drained

1/4 cup olives, pitted and chopped

1/3 cup basil pesto

1 tbsp fresh dill, chopped

1/4 cup capers

1 tsp paprika

1/4 tsp salt

Directions:

1.Season salmon with paprika and salt. Place the cooking tray in the air fryer basket. Place piece of parchment paper into the air fryer basket.

2.Select Bake mode. Set time to 20 minutes and temperature 400 F then press START.

3.The air fryer display will prompt you to ADD FOOD once the temperature is reached then place salmon in the air fryer basket and top with remaining ingredients. Serve and enjoy.

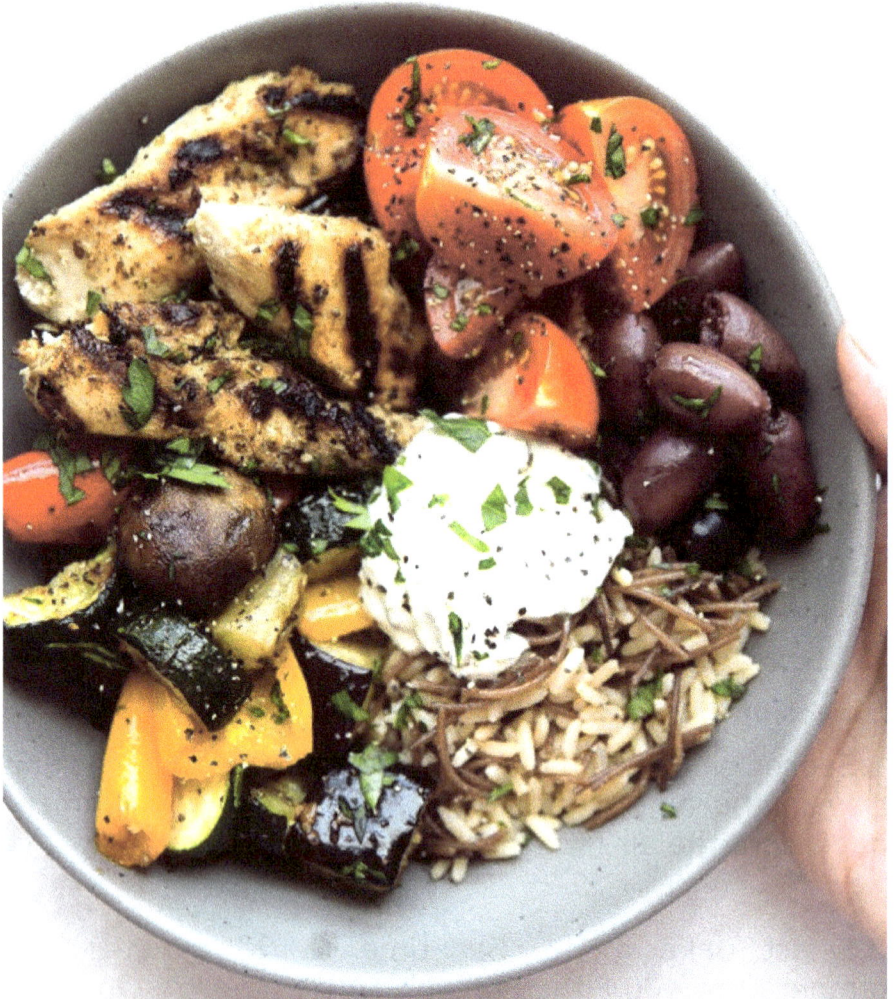

White Fish Fillet with Roasted Pepper

Preparation Time:

10 minutes

Cooking Time:

30 minutes

Serve: 1

Ingredients:

8 oz frozen white fish fillet

1/2 tsp Italian seasoning

1 1/2 tbsp butter, melted

 1 tbsp lemon juice

1 tbsp fresh parsley, chopped

1 tbsp roasted red bell pepper, diced

Directions:

1.Place the fish fillet in a baking dish. Drizzle butter and lemon juice over fish.

2.Sprinkle with Italian seasoning. Top with roasted bell pepper and parsley. Select Bake mode.

3.Set time to 30 minutes and temperature 400 F then press START.

4.The air fryer display will prompt you to ADD FOOD once the temperature is reached then place the baking dish in the air fryer basket. Serve and enjoy

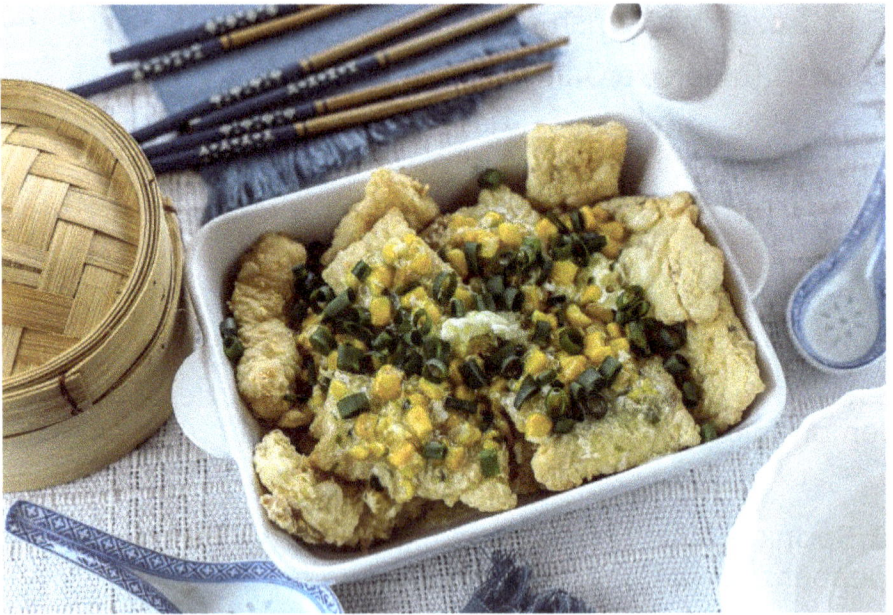

Rosemary Basil Salmon

Preparation Time:

10 minutes

Cooking Time:

15 minutes

Serve: 4

Ingredients:

1 lbs salmon, cut into

4 pieces 1 tbsp olive oil

1/2 tbsp dried rosemary

1/4 tsp dried basil

1 tbsp dried chives

Pepper Salt

Directions:

1.Mix together olive oil, basil, chives, and rosemary. Brush salmon with oil mixture.

2.Select Air Fry mode. Set time to 15 minutes and temperature 400 F then press START.

3.The air fryer display will prompt you to ADD FOOD once the temperature is reached then place salmon pieces in the air fryer basket. Serve and enjoy.

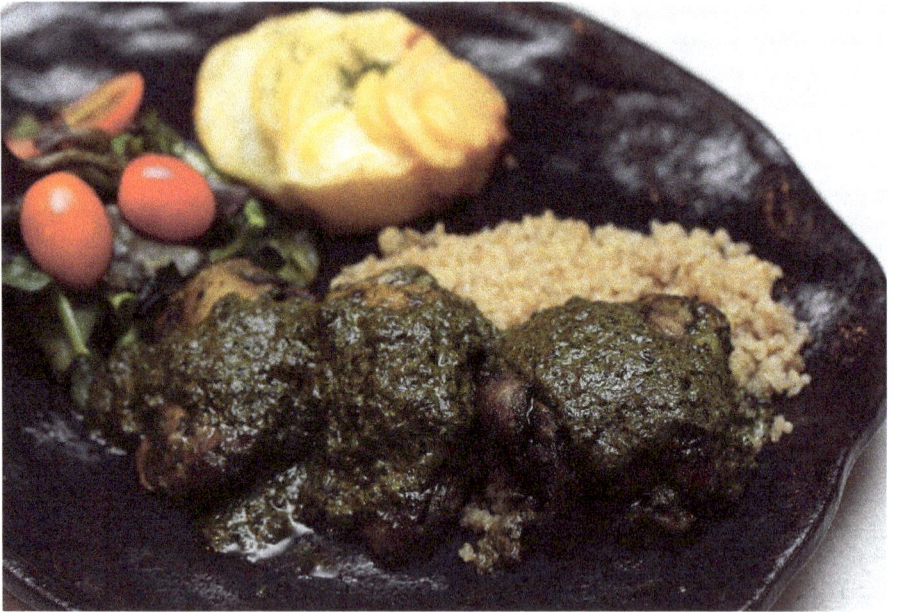

Tomato Basil Fish Fillets

Preparation Time:

10 minutes

Cooking Time:

20 minutes

Serve: 2

Ingredients:

2 salmon fillets

1 tomato, sliced

1 tbsp dried basil

2 tbsp parmesan cheese, grated

1 tbsp olive oil

Directions:

1.Place salmon fillets in the baking dish. Sprinkle basil on top of salmon fillets. Arrange tomato slices on top of salmon fillets.

2.Drizzle with oil and sprinkle cheese on top. Select Bake mode. Set time to 20 minutes and temperature 375 F then press START.

3.The air fryer display will prompt you to ADD FOOD once the temperature is reached then place the baking dish in the air fryer basket. Serve and enjoy.

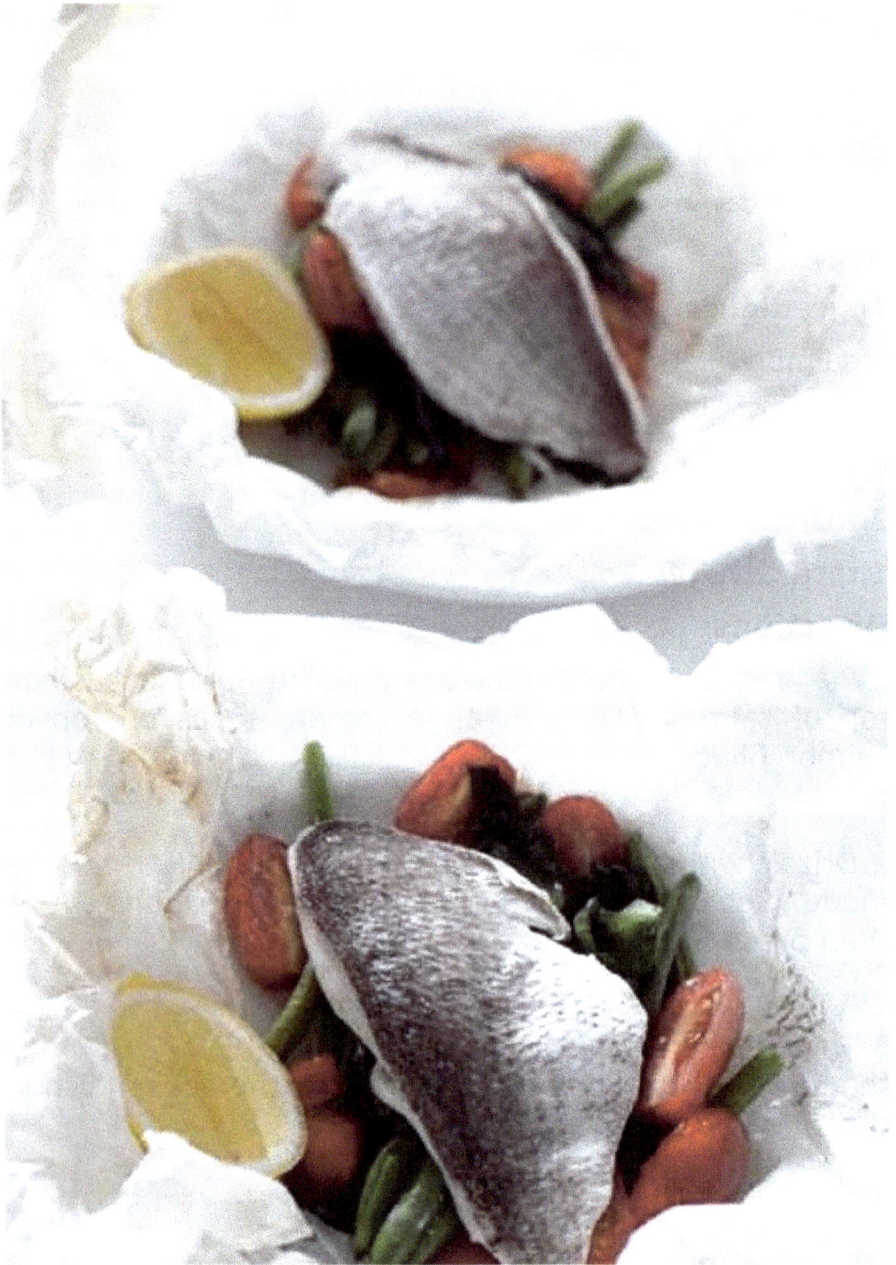